"I love this book! The integrity of the information is rock solid. The recipes are simple, practical, nourishing, and very satisfying. Learning to cook with the seasons is a great way to reconnect with nature and the pulse of life. I especially enjoyed the sea vegetable dishes that provide trace elements missing from the Western diet."

—EDWARD BAUMAN, Med, PhD, Director, Bauman College:
Holistic Nutrition and Culinary Arts, Penngrove, CA

The Everything® Guide to Macrobiotics is as comprehensive as its title suggests. Julie's tips are easy to follow and put into practical use in one's daily regimen. It is especially useful for beginners, but also as a refresher for old-timers. I recommend this book to everyone who wants to live and eat in a healthy and happy macrobiotic way."

—SANAE SUZUKI, Author, *Love, Sanae, Healing Vegan
Macrobiotic Cooking*, and Co-owner of Seed,
Vegan Macrobiotic Kitchen in Venice, CA

The Everything® Guide to Macrobiotics is the perfect book for anyone interested in enhancing their wellness naturally through preparing common healthy foods; it's easy to follow, yet offers new, innovative, and practical ideas for parents and people with busy lives. I highly recommend this valuable book."

—MICHAEL REED GACH, PhD, Acupressure.com Producer
and Bestselling Author of *Acupressure's Potent Points*
and *Acupressure for Emotional Healing*

The Everything® Guide to Macrobiotics is an easy-to-read, articulate macrobiotic primer with seasonal wisdom and delicious recipes from the friendly voice of Julie S. Ong. Definitely worth a good chew!"

—VERNE VARONA, Author, *Macrobiotics for Dummies*

THE
EVERYTHING®
GUIDE TO MACROBIOTICS

Dear Reader,

The Everything® Guide to Macrobiotics is a cookbook that represents my macrobiotic and spiritual journey so far. Through macrobiotics, balance, and spirituality, I have changed my lifestyle, and it has changed me in return. I feel free, happy, and peaceful. To be connected to my source, my spirit, my inspiration, is to find my center, my balance with the universe. I am so happy, my heart wants to burst open and embrace the universe.

I want you to share the joy of finding your center. In this book, some foods may be more familiar to you than others. I encourage you to explore the energetic components of a wide range of foods. Include healing foods that are more aligned with your cultural traditions. This will help you connect to spirit through your food source.

I couldn't be more pleased to share this knowledge with you, and I hope you enjoy your journey into macrobiotics. . . .

Happy cooking!

Julie S. Ong

Welcome to the EVERYTHING® Series!

These handy, accessible books give you all you need to tackle a difficult project, gain a new hobby, comprehend a fascinating topic, prepare for an exam, or even brush up on something you learned back in school but have since forgotten.

You can choose to read an Everything® book from cover to cover or just pick out the information you want from our four useful boxes: e-questions, e-facts, e-alerts, and e-ssentials.

We give you everything you need to know on the subject, but throw in a lot of fun stuff along the way, too.

We now have more than 400 Everything® books in print, spanning such wide-ranging categories as weddings, pregnancy, cooking, music instruction, foreign language, crafts, pets, New Age, and so much more. When you're done reading them all, you can finally say you know Everything®!

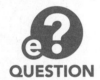
QUESTION
Answers to common questions

FACT
Important snippets of information

ALERT
Urgent warnings

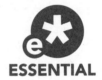
ESSENTIAL
Quick handy tips

PUBLISHER Karen Cooper

DIRECTOR OF ACQUISITIONS AND INNOVATION Paula Munier

MANAGING EDITOR, EVERYTHING® SERIES Lisa Laing

COPY CHIEF Casey Ebert

ACQUISITIONS EDITOR Katrina Schroeder

ASSOCIATE DEVELOPMENT EDITOR Hillary Thompson

EDITORIAL ASSISTANT Ross Weisman

EVERYTHING® SERIES COVER DESIGNER Erin Alexander

LAYOUT DESIGNERS Colleen Cunningham, Elisabeth Lariviere, Ashley Vierra, Denise Wallace

Visit the entire Everything® series at *www.everything.com*

THE
EVERYTHING®
GUIDE TO MACROBIOTICS

A practical introduction to the macrobiotic
lifestyle—and how it can work for you

Julie S. Ong with Lorena Novak Bull, RD

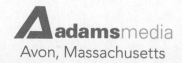
Avon, Massachusetts

This book is dedicated to my grandmother,
who is my greatest Spiritual Guide.

An Everything® Series Book.
Everything® and everything.com® are registered trademarks of F+W Media, Inc.

Published by Adams Media, a division of F+W Media, Inc.
57 Littlefield Street, Avon, MA 02322 U.S.A.
www.adamsmedia.com

ISBN 10: 1-4405-0371-0
ISBN 13: 978-1-4405-0371-9
eISBN 10: 1-4405-0372-9
eISBN 13: 978-1-4405-0372-6

Printed in the United States of America.

10 9 8 7 6 5 4 3 2 1

Library of Congress Cataloging-in-Publication Data
is available from the publisher.

This publication is designed to provide accurate and authoritative information with regard to the subject matter covered. It is sold with the understanding that the publisher is not engaged in rendering legal, accounting, or other professional advice. If legal advice or other expert assistance is required, the services of a competent professional person should be sought.

—From a *Declaration of Principles* jointly adopted by a Committee of the American Bar Association and a Committee of Publishers and Associations

Many of the designations used by manufacturers and sellers to distinguish their products are claimed as trademarks. Where those designations appear in this book and Adams Media was aware of a trademark claim, the designations have been printed with initial capital letters.

The Everything® Guide to Macrobiotics is intended as a reference volume only, not as a medical manual. In light of the complex, individual, and specific nature of health problems, this book is not intended to replace professional medical advice. The ideas, procedures, and suggestions in this book are intended to supplement, not replace, the advice of a trained medical professional. Consult your physician before adopting the suggestions in this book, as well as about any condition that may require diagnosis or medical attention. The author and publisher disclaim any liability arising directly or indirectly from the use of this book.

This book is available at quantity discounts for bulk purchases.
For information, please call 1-800-289-0963.

Contents

Acknowledgments

Setting out on a spiritual path attracts loving companions who provide support along the way. My steps have been blessed with very special relationships that have guided me toward conscious awakening. I am eternally grateful for and humbled by each person's contribution in my life.

My constant companion is Spirit, who is my greatest strength and support. Each day reminds me of Spirit's eternal love and grace. It was through divine inspiration that this book was written, and that brings me deeper into my own authentic self.

My friends during the creative process of this book are too numerous to mention. However, there are a few who not only supported this endeavor, but who guided me toward greater self-awareness.

I give great thanks to my friend Dave Cunningham of FrontRunnersLLC. com for his love and encouragement, which guided me forward when I felt overwhelmed.

I am also grateful to Carolyn Wilson-Elliott of QuantumSpirit.net for her wisdom and feedback as each chapter was blossoming. Her unwavering support reminds me to express gratitude for creative energies in the universal dance of life.

I wish to thank the following people for their love and support in holding my vision: Sherry Hudson, of DeliberateSuccess.com; Deborah Ivanoff, of Answering-the-Sacred.com; and Carole Yeend, of True Vibrations. It is an honor to have the opportunity to co-create with such blessed beings.

I also wish to thank my macrobiotic friends for mirroring my truth and holding my hand on our universal journey.

Finally, I am blessed to have my sister, Kathy, and my mother, Lily, by my side, providing continuous gifts of love.

Introduction

MACROBIOTICS IS A WAY of living in harmony with the present moment—with your present health condition, your present lifestyle, and your present needs and desires. When your health and lifestyle change, you evolve and adjust along with your flexible needs and desires. You incorporate healthier ways of living, because they closely match the priorities in your life in this present moment. As you intentionally choose your path, you experience the healing result that you desire. Your inner awareness guides you to listen to your body and balance your present needs in the moment. The key word here is "you." Everyone is unique. Everyone finds his or her own sense of harmony in the present moment.

The intention of this book is to help you connect with nature and live a macrobiotic life through mindful food choices. Trusting your intuition will cultivate your connection with your spirit. You will be guided toward a life filled with happiness, freedom, and peace. As your heart opens in a deep and enduring way, this feeling of balance and harmony becomes normal. This feeling becomes the standard for which you strive to bring about continuing health, one baby step at a time.

Macrobiotics is an ancient art of living that is rooted in a profound understanding of the laws and patterns of nature, as applied to the human body. This understanding sees the human body as an integral part of the natural world. Through food, you connect with your spiritual nature and open yourself up to natural healing. Macrobiotics is about living in harmony with nature and trusting your intuition. This Zen perspective incorporates seasonal, locally grown, and energetically balanced foods into your life. The word "macrobiotics" literally means "large life" ("macro" means "large or great" and "bio" means "life").

Along with a macrobiotic diet, adjustments in ways of living can make a difference in balancing health on all levels. This is *wholistic* living, and goes one step further than holistic medicine, which treats the mind and body through complementary health care. (The "w" is inserted to distinguish the broader experience of *wholistic* living from the common application of holistic therapy.) When you understand the energy of foods and how to balance this energy, you can experience this *wholistic*, or whole, way of living.

In this book, you will learn how diet affects your physical body and emotions and how you can balance your health condition and lifestyle with natural healing foods. Nothing is excluded from the macrobiotic diet. Even extreme foods, if balanced, can be healing. More specifically, it is about choosing foods that support and harmonize your dynamic changing health condition. Adjusting your cooking according to the seasons provides the foundational blueprint (or recipe) for living a long life from a more insightful perspective.

Ancient cultures intuitively knew how to balance the energy of food with the seasons to extend their life through natural means. Natural healers, such as grandmothers and wise elders, through daily meals as well as herbal teas and rich mineral broths, knew how to live in harmony with nature. Every tradition has a special healing dish that has been passed on from one generation to the next. Strengthening bone soups were lovingly prepared by Hungarian grandmothers for use after childbirth. Cleansing bitter teas with hints of licorice were brewed by Chinese fathers for use as cold remedies. These were special "chicken soup–like" home remedies, designed to carry a particular healing aspect other than calories, carbohydrates, and vitamins. This healing essence of food can nourish, heal, and harmonize every aspect of the body, mind, emotion, and spirit.

Traditional healing dishes that are cooked according to the seasons imbibe this essence of "soul food."

Vibrant, energetically balanced food nourishes body, mind, and spirit; it balances emotions and contributes to overall health and well being. Macrobiotics can help you develop this connection with food, an intimate relationship that enhances your intuition and brings you to the present moment.

CHAPTER 1

Introduction to Macrobiotics

More than a diet, macrobiotics is a *wholistic* way of living that ensures everlasting peace and freedom. It is a way of living in harmony with the natural order by following the principles and laws of the universe. When your energy is balanced and harmonious, true health radiates from the inside out. Imagine having a blissful smile on your face, sparkling eyes, youthful energy, a heart full of joy and gratitude, a peaceful mind, and a free spirit. Whatever your dream, with macrobiotics, you can create a life you truly love.

What Is Macrobiotics?

Macrobiotics (macro = large or great, bios = life) is based on the Far Eastern concept of cultivating health and longevity by balancing your unique energy with the natural order. The natural order includes circulating life energy, your moods, spirit, and nature. The macrobiotic path includes eating seasonal, locally grown, and energetically balanced foods. Besides providing important nutrients, such as protein, carbohydrates, vitamins, and minerals, food is important for healthy organ and immune function and in maintaining overall energetic balance in the body.

Chi

The true foundation of macrobiotics is circulating life energy, called *chi* in Chinese. Chi is thought to be the force that animates and enlightens all things. Macrobiotics balances your current health condition with certain healing foods based on their chi or energy signatures, rather than solely on their nutritional content. This food may come in the form of biological foods, such as plants and animals, or elements, such as air, water, and inorganic salts. Since life is dependent on energy, your body converts chi in your food into heat or uses it for other processes.

ESSENTIAL

Acupressure is another ancient healing art that activates chi to bring organ systems back to harmony. It uses fingers to press key points on meridians to engage circulating chi for self-healing. Acupressure and acupuncture use the same points, but acupressure uses fingers, while acupuncture uses needles to pinpoint areas of blocked energy.

Meridians

In the human body, chi flows through energy channels, or pathways, called meridians. Meridians form an energy network that connects all organ systems in the body. Chi travels through this network to various organs, which transmit messages to each other. Because this energy network links meridians and all parts of the body with each other, circulating chi unifies the body as a whole. Blockages in meridians can cause problems in organs. So keeping the meridians clear is important for proper function of the body's processes.

Function of Meridians

Meridians reflect and react to the energetic changes of environmental conditions, such as seasons, time of day, and climate. A functional meridian system manifests as a healthy body in a state of homeostasis, a dynamic yet balanced condition of harmonious energies. Because meridians respond to and transmit information, they have the ability to bring healing energy to many areas of the body. At certain locations along the meridian, the energy signature of specific healing foods can enhance or modify the flow of chi. This can create physical, mental, emotional, and spiritual changes as chi circulates, so that healing occurs in multiple dimensions.

FACT

Besides macrobiotics, tai chi is an ancient Chinese art that also induces a state of relaxation and calm. It uses graceful, flowing dancelike movements that improve energy, strength, and flexibility. Used as a mind-body practice, tai chi can help relieve anxiety and depression, improve balance and coordination, lower blood pressure, and reduce the number of falls in the elderly.

Excessive Versus Deficient Chi

Meridians and their linked organ systems are the basis for identifying the root cause of dis-eases and what foods heal them. The hyphenated variation of "disease" suggests that the natural state of "ease" (chi) is imbalanced or disrupted. For clarity, the term "disease" (without the hyphen) will be used in this book. Diseases fall into one of two categories: those resulting from overactive (excessive) energy or those resulting from underactive (deficient) energy. Healing foods balance excessive energy by calming or dispersing this energy in an organ system. Conversely, healing foods balance deficient energy through activating or supplying energy to an organ system.

"Chi stagnation" is a form of excessive energy in the body. In chi stagnation, energy and information is prevented from traveling to and from its destination. If chi stagnates in a meridian for too long, the meridian can become blocked and eventually manifest as disease. Stagnated organs can also become vulnerable to external pathogens. So freely flowing chi through meridians and organs is the foundation for a strong healthy body. Another energy function problem is an overall "chi deficiency," in which an organ system has weak or deficient chi. In this case, the organ system needs to be strengthened to build up chi, which in turn builds up the body overall.

Yin and Yang

In macrobiotics, the balance of opposite but complementary forms of life energy, or chi, in the body is the foundation for good health. Everything is composed of these two complementary opposite energies: One energy is called "yin" and the other is called "yang." Never separate, neither energy can exist without the other. These energies are intertwined and dependent on each other, rather than antagonistic. This interconnectedness can be seen in the ancient yin/yang symbol, in which each section contains the energy of the other. Additionally, nothing is ever yin or yang alone; it is always yin or yang in relation to something else. For instance, noon is yang in relation to morning, which is more yin. However, morning is yang compared to night, which is more yin.

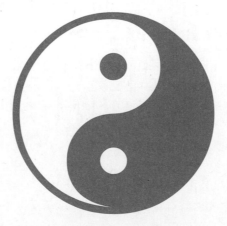

Yin Yang Symbol

▼ **TABLE 1-1: CHARACTERISTICS OF YIN AND YANG**

Yin	Yang
Centrifugal	Centripetal
Expansion	Contraction
Letting go	Gathering and pulling in
Upward	Downward
Outward	Inward
Lighter	Heavier
Wetter	Drier
Less dense	Denser
Larger	Smaller
Softer	Harder

Yin and yang exist in harmony and dynamic change, not just static balance. There is a continuous, natural balance that exists between these energies. They exist in a state of energetic homeostasis; when one expands, the other contracts. A healthy body is in harmony not only internally within the body itself, but also externally, in relationship with the natural order of the universe. So, when nature's chi adjusts itself each season, a person's internal chi acclimates automatically. Any time chi is out of harmony, either within or without, disease is the result.

ESSENTIAL

The kinds of foods you eat can affect your mental health. Eating excess contracting (yang) foods creates paranoia and a tendency to hold on to the past. On the contrary, eating a more ungrounded (yin) diet results in schizophrenia and focusing too far forward into the future.

What Is a Balanced Meal?

A balanced macrobiotic meal may include one dish or several dishes. The main goal in designing a macrobiotic meal is to create harmonious balance of all energies on the plate. These energies include color, taste, texture, flavor, and shapes of food. For example, brown rice alone is not a macrobiotic meal. The energy of brown rice is not balanced by itself. But, sprinkling roasted sesame salt (gomashio) on top balances bitter flavor with the sweetness in the rice, with the added benefit of aiding digestion. Garnishes are also used to help balance energies in a macrobiotic meal. Pungent scallions provide yin energy to balance yang foods, such as fish (and also help dissolve oils). Although they did not intellectually understand the principles of yin and yang (macrobiotics), traditional cultures were intimately connected with the land, seasons, and cycles. They intuitively knew how to balance energies in foods. For example:

- Yang salty, oily fish and chips were often served with yin vinegar or lemon.
- Yang turkey was combined with yin cranberry sauce.
- A Reuben sandwich was made with acidic yang corned beef and alkalinizing yin sauerkraut.
- Yang egg omelets were made with yin tomatoes or ketchup.
- Yang heavy, dense hamburgers were served with pungent raw onion or yin ketchup.
- Yang fatty, dense steak was seasoned with yin pepper.

FACT

Traditional cultures intuitively knew how to eat according to the seasons and climate. The Inuit consume foods that are hunted, fished, and gathered locally. Their diet consists mainly of walrus, seal, whale, polar bear, and fireweed. This mostly yang meat diet is ideal for keeping the body warm, strong, fit, and healthy in the Arctic's cold yin climate.

Chapter 4 contains an overview of the standard macrobiotic diet and the choice of foods, condiments, seasonings, and so on. Healing foods that balance one person's energy may not work for someone else. Adjustments must be made to the standard macrobiotic diet based on your changing needs, including season and climate. Chapter 2 discusses how to make adjustments in cooking based on season and climate.

By using macrobiotic principles, you can learn the art of macrobiotic cooking. (Refer to Chapter 3 for guidelines on balancing macrobiotic meals.) Eventually, your intuition will guide you in balancing your condition with specific foods for healing on many levels—physical, mental, emotional, and spiritual.

Balanced Versus Extreme Foods

Throughout history, ancient cultures have looked to cereal grains as their main source of food. Indeed, the basis of the standard macrobiotic diet is whole grains, especially brown rice, which contains the most ideal ratio of basic nutrients for humans.

Whole Grains

Whole grains are living foods that are intact and still contain the nutritious bran and germ portions. You know they are alive because a new plant sprouts from the seed (grain). This means that, besides being nutritious and high in fiber, this living chi increases your own vitality.

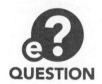

QUESTION

Can I eat sprouted grains instead of cooking them?
The process of sprouting changes complex carbohydrates into simple sugars. These simple sugars make sprouted grains more yin than whole cooked grains. In hot climates, sprouted grains, along with raw foods, are appropriate in salads to balance yang atmospheric energy. However, overconsumption of these cooling foods can deplete energy and weaken your body.

Whole grains also contain complex carbohydrates (with intact fiber), which break down slowly in the body, keeping blood sugar levels steady. However, refined grains and white flour products are polished and contain only the endosperm. Besides lacking nutrients and fiber, they are composed of simple sugars, which spike blood sugar levels during digestion.

Cracked grains, like rolled oats, and whole grain flour products (whole grain bread) are also considered to have deficient energy compared to that of intact whole grains, since cracked and milled grains are no longer alive. Additionally, high heat used in the milling process even destroys the nutritional value of whole grains. Whole grain diets may reduce the risks of heart disease, some cancers, and type-2 diabetes, and may help with weight management.

Extreme Yang Foods

Relative to balanced foods, yang foods have gathering energy, which stabilizes the body and mind. These foods gather nutrients into the system, which creates strength, firmness, and hardness. The body becomes dense, solid, and grounded. However, overconsumption of extreme yang foods, such as meat and cheese, can lead to stagnation and congestion along with rigid thinking. This condition may lead to cravings for yin foods, such as sugar, from the other extreme for balance.

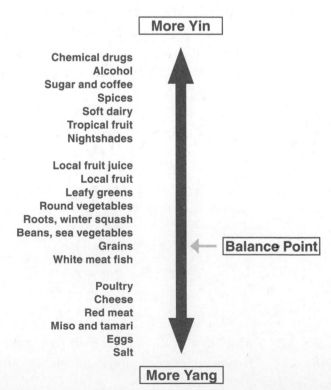

More Yin

Chemical drugs
Alcohol
Sugar and coffee
Spices
Soft dairy
Tropical fruit
Nightshades

Local fruit juice
Local fruit
Leafy greens
Round vegetables
Roots, winter squash
Beans, sea vegetables
Grains
White meat fish

Poultry
Cheese
Red meat
Miso and tamari
Eggs
Salt

← Balance Point

More Yang

Yin and Yang Balance Chart

Extreme Yin Foods	Standard Macrobiotic Diet	Extreme Yang Foods
Chemical drugs	Local fruit juice	Poultry
Alcohol	Local fruit	Cheese
Sugar and coffee	Leafy greens	Red meat
Spices	Round vegetables	Miso and tamari
Soft dairy	Roots, winter squash	Eggs
Tropical fruit	Beans, sea vegetables	Salt
Nightshades	Grains	
	White meat fish	

ESSENTIAL

In Japanese, *sanpaku* means "three whites," indicating an imbalanced nervous system. Someone with *yin sanpaku* eyes is vulnerable to danger from the outside world. White that shows below the iris is caused by overconsumption of yin foods. However, someone with *yang sanpaku* eyes is prone to violence within themselves. White that shows above the iris is caused by excessive intake of yang foods.

Extreme Yin Foods

Compared to balanced foods, yin foods activate the body and mind. These foods release energy and nutrients into the system, which creates relaxation. The body becomes softer, lighter, and more open. Extreme yin foods, however, break down yang areas of the body. Long time meat eaters often become attracted to raw foods, since the cooling yin nature of raw foods can help break up and disperse hard yang areas of the body. However, vegans can actually become weak on a diet solely of yin foods, since too much energy is dispersed without grounding yang energy to balance it. Overconsumption of extreme yin foods can lead to cravings for yang foods of the opposite extreme for balance.

How Food Affects Moods

Emotional symptoms associated with health difficulties can be additional signals of imbalance. Each organ is related to an emotion, which can be altered by changing the energy of your body through the kinds of foods you eat. If your body is blocked from mucous-causing foods (like dairy and white flour products), organs become stagnated as toxins accumulate, resulting in extreme emotions. For example, when the liver is toxic from overconsumption of alcohol, anger or shouting is an emotional discharge. Chapter 2 will discuss specific foods and cooking styles that nourish and support each organ.

Organs and Traditional Chinese Medicine

In contrast to the Western view, traditional Chinese medicine (TCM) describes organ systems as a spectrum of body and mind interrelationships and connections rather than anatomical organs. Because TCM is *wholistic*, organs are described in relationship to other organ systems, going beyond just their physiology. A capital letter distinguishes TCM organ systems from Western organs. In this book, organs will not be capitalized, for clarity.

▼   TABLE 1-3: ORGANS AND EMOTIONAL HEALTH

Organ	Imbalanced Emotion	Balanced Emotion
Liver	Anger, shouting	Kindness, patience
Heart	Anxiety, excessive talking	Joy
Spleen	Worry	Sympathy, compassion
Lung	Depression, sadness	Sense of worthiness
Kidney	Fear, insecurity	Courage

Emotions of the Liver

A healthy liver expresses emotions of patience and kindness. An imbalance in liver energy, however, results in emotions of anger or impatience being released. In the opposite way, unexpressed or excessive emotions, such as depression or long-term frustration, can create an imbalance in the liver. The-best case scenario, then, is a peaceful lifestyle and balanced emotional state, which are both important for healthy liver function.

Upward growing vegetables, such as sprouts, contain the same energetic frequency as the liver to nourish and support the detoxification and discharge of emotional stagnation. Also, downward growing vegetables, such as kuzu root and carrots, can counterbalance overly active emotion (anger) in the liver.

Emotions of the Heart

Heart health is intimately connected with the mind and emotions. Tuning in to your intuition can give you clues as to the condition of your heart. A healthy, peaceful heart elicits feelings of joy and happiness. However, excessive laughter suggests a heart that is overactive and unbalanced. On the flip side, factors like depression, anxiety, or no laughter at all may be strong predictors of heart problems. Symptomatic of underlying problems, longtime dysfunctional emotional states can be accurate indicators of physical heart conditions. So physical heart disease may be the manifestation of suppressed emotions that appear in your body as physical symptoms.

FACT

Broken heart syndrome is a kind of nonischemic cardiomyopathy in which the heart muscle becomes weakened from traumatic emotional or physical stress. Sudden grief can release a flood of stress hormones that cause heart spasms that mimic a heart attack. However, because the heart is not permanently damaged, recovery rates for broken heart syndrome are faster than for a heart attack.

Leafy greens, which have upward rising and expansive chi, support the upper part of the body, such as the heart. Broad leafy greens especially help to open and expand the heart's capacity for feeling joy and happiness. Foods that have downward gathering chi, such as the sea vegetable hijiki and roots, can also help ground an overly emotional heart.

Emotions of the Spleen

Healthy expressions of sympathy and compassion for yourself and others can strengthen your spleen energy. However, obsession, anxiety, worry, and brooding are imbalanced emotions related to a depleted spleen. Indulging in these emotions weakens digestion to the point of decreased appetite, poor digestion, bloating, gas, and ulcers.

Foods that are mildly sweet, such as butternut squash, have relaxing energy. This relaxing chi nourishes the spleen's capacity for sympathy and compassion. These feelings can be expressed as openness to the sweetness in life.

Emotions of the Lung

Emotions associated with balanced lung function are righteousness, surrender, letting go, and emptiness. This makes sense as the process of surrender is one of connecting with your breath, so that you can release one breath before you receive another. However, the emotions associated with deficient lung chi are sadness, grief, and sorrow. Suppression of these emotions restricts lung function, leading to fatigue, depression, and weakened immune system.

Some cosmetics and perfumes contain toxic chemical fragrances that, when breathed in, can damage lung and brain cells. Instead, choose "green" products, which are environmentally safe and made from organic ingredients. Also, walk outside for half an hour daily to improve your blood and lymph circulation, cleanse your lungs, and lift your spirits.

Foods that nourish the lung's capacity to let go and surrender have a downward, gathering energy, such as brown rice, lotus root, and burdock root.

Emotions of the Kidney

When kidney chi is balanced, determination and will are strong. This can manifest as mental strength, focus, and drive to achieve goals. However, blocked kidney chi can express the emotion of fear. Conversely, fear can weaken the kidney if prolonged. In children, fear can manifest as bed wetting, and in adults, it can result in anxiety and heart troubles.

Foods that support the kidney's capacity for motivation and mental focus have deeply concentrated energy, such as dried roots.

Connection with Nature

Spiritual development plays an important role in transformational healing. Ancient masters understood the multidimensional process of healing, in which balance and harmony occurs in mind, body, emotions, and spirit. They recognized that this harmonious healing process extends to an individual's relationship with nature as well.

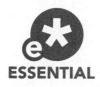

ESSENTIAL

The founder of macrobiotics, George Ohsawa, recognized an ancient wisdom shared by sages. He realized that the underlying cause of disease was arrogance itself, or treating the body as if it existed independently from nature. Indeed, limited thought patterns can create resistance in the body and manifest as disease. However, softening and opening up to unlimited potential creates healing and wholeness.

Energetically Balanced Foods

Your energetic body is fluid and changing in response to the subtle frequencies of the universe. If your meridians are blocked, growth of the body is stunted and illness develops. Healthy food helps to unblock and nourish the meridians, so that you can receive life energy and live in harmony with nature and the universe.

Spiritual Essence of Food

An energetically balanced diet can also open your meridians and strengthen your spiritual energy. This allows your intuition to become stronger. Physical pain can be an indication that spiritual energy is deficient and meridians are blocked. If your energy is out of alignment with nature, your body can become weak and vulnerable to attack from viruses and bacteria. Likewise, your intuition can also become weak and this makes you vulnerable to dangerous situations. When you live in harmony with the natural order by eating energetically balanced foods, you strengthen your spiritual essence and experience a strong connection with nature and the universe.

CHAPTER 2

Cooking According to the Seasons

As each season unfolds, plants receive nourishment from the natural elemental forces of sun, wind, rain, and soil. Growth rings in the trunks of giant Sequoias record seasonal activity that has affected their growth. Likewise, growing tissues in your body record areas of disrupted chi, which is naturally fluid and changing in response to seasonal activity. If your meridians are blocked from eating mucous-causing food, your body becomes stagnant and illness develops. However, eating seasonal food cleanses and nourishes these energy channels, and cooking food according to the seasons maximizes the chi available for your body to heal.

Spring Energy

If you understand spring energy, you can balance macrobiotic cooking to achieve peace and better health. For many people, spring means the end of winter, a promise of summer and vacation, baseball games, and being outdoors. It is a celebration of bright yellow daffodils, crocuses emerging from the earth, people walking outside, buds on the trees, little patches of melting snow, and people smiling. Plant energy, along with atmospheric energy, rises upward and new growth appears as weather becomes warmer. Spring, with its upward, rising energy, is related to the wood element.

FACT

In traditional Chinese medicine, organs are never seen as just physical organs. Each organ also corresponds to innumerable qualities, such as body tissue, sense organ, emotion, taste, sound, season, time of day, element, and direction. These associated qualities provide healthcare practitioners with a foundation for understanding, diagnosing, and treating disease.

The vital organ most associated with spring is the liver, along with its paired organ, the gallbladder, which are both supported by foods that have rising, upward energy. Hours when these organs are most active are between 1:00 AM and 3:00 AM for liver and 11:00 PM and 1:00 AM for gallbladder.

▼ **TABLE 2-1: ENERGY AND VEGETABLES OF THE SEASONS**

Organs	Energy	Season	Taste	Vegetable
Liver, gallbladder	Upward	Spring	Sour	Sprouts and upward growing plants
Heart, small intestine	Very active	Summer	Bitter	Large leafy greens
Spleen, pancreas, stomach	Downward	Late summer	Sweet	Ground or round plants

Organs	Energy	Season	Taste	Vegetable
Lungs, large intestine	Solidified	Autumn	Pungent	Root vegetables
Kidneys, bladder	Floating	Winter	Salty	Root plants, dried roots

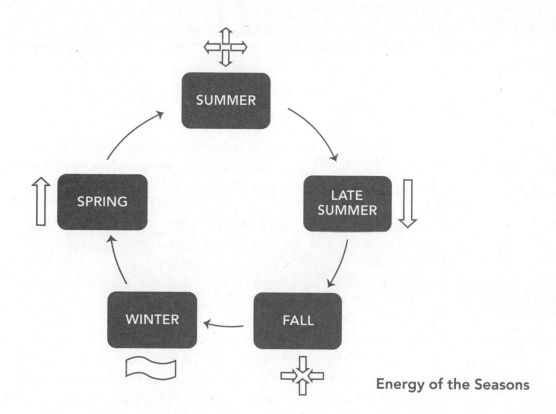

Energy of the Seasons

Functions of the Liver

The liver's functions harmonize with the upward, rising activity of spring. The liver regulates the free and easy movement of energy (chi) in the body and stores and controls the blood. It also plays an important role in the health of the eyes, nails, ligaments, and tendons.

Controls Chi

The first of the liver's functions is to ensure the free and easy movement of chi in the body. In the spring, when energy is rising, excess liver energy rises too quickly, which may cause headaches or migraines at the top of the head where the liver energy pathway (or meridian) flows. Dizziness and hypertension can also occur as energy rises in spring, along with mood swings and excessive emotional reactions.

Stores and Circulates Blood

Another important function of the liver is to store blood at rest and send blood into the circulatory system during activity. Not only is this function important for providing nourishment to other organs, but it is also important in a woman's health to regulate the menstrual blood flow for regular, pain-free menstrual cycles.

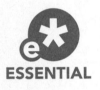

ESSENTIAL

In traditional Chinese medicine, organs work together in pairs in organ systems. This interaction of organ partners determines how well the body functions as a whole. The yang organ is solid and dense (liver), while its yin partner is hollow (gallbladder). The focus is on the solid yang organ, since it has more gathering energy, which is the source for chi in the organ system.

However, when the liver is malfunctioning, a woman may experience irregular periods, PMS, cramps, breast pain, and headaches or migraines. The uterus itself is particularly dependent on proper liver function and free flowing movement of chi and blood. If there is blockage of chi, a build-up of fibroids and lumps can occur in the breasts and uterus that can develop into cancer.

Opens into the Eyes

The eyes are the opening to the liver. Signs of unbalanced liver chi appear as problems in the eyes, since a branch of the liver meridian flows into the eyes. Deficient liver chi can cause blurred vision, dry or swollen eyes, and floaters. Overuse of the eyes can also lead to deficient liver chi.

Maintains Nails

Fingernails and toenails are also under the influence of the liver. Signs of poor nourishment and deficient liver chi can show up as weak nails: pale, brittle, chipped, ridges, fungus, or missing the half moon at the base.

Governs Ligaments and Tendons

Areas of the body that are also influenced by liver function are tendons and ligaments. Blood deficiency in these areas can create spasms or sluggish movement in the joints. The opposite is also true: Overworking your joints and ligaments through excess exercise can weaken the liver, which must increase blood flow to restore them. Deficient liver energy has an impact on a woman's health, as excessive exercise can cause a woman's menstrual flow to cease.

ALERT

A direct correlation has been found between fibroids and xenoestrogens, which are estrogen-like compounds in food and pesticides. Mimicking the body's hormones, xenoestrogens can contribute to increased estrogen levels, triggering fibroid growth spurts. Eating foods high on the food chain, such as meat, fish, and dairy products, can increase exposure to these non-biodegradable hormones.

Functions of the Gallbladder

The gallbladder functions to store bile created by the liver and excrete this bile into the duodenum. Bile helps dissolve fats that enter the digestive system. If gallstones block the passage from the gallbladder to the duodenum, bile goes instead into the blood, making the skin yellow-green.

Cooking for Spring

The essence of each food harmonizes the healing energy of a particular organ, or even several organs, restoring balance to a weakened organ system. Including seasonal organic foods in your diet strengthens the corresponding organ system for a particular season. Foods that especially nurture liver and gallbladder are those with upward, growing spring energy, such as barley, sprouts, and leeks. Sour taste is associated with spring, and sour foods, such as umeboshi plum and lemon, help the liver discharge excess oily foods from winter cooking. Upward-growing shiitake mushrooms also dissolve fat in the liver, relaxing a contracted body to improve the free and easy movement of chi. Lightly cooked dishes and less oil encourage energy to move upward, helping to dissolve stagnation in the body. Spring cooking styles include:

- Blanching
- Boiled grains
- Quick marinated pickles
- Quick pressed salad
- Quick sauté

▼ **TABLE 2-2: FOODS THAT SUPPORT LIVER ENERGY**

Grains	Beans	Vegetables	Sea Vegetable	Fruit
Barley, hato mugi, oats, rye, wheat	Edamame, lentils, peas	Upward growing plants (celery, chives, spring greens, green beans, leeks, mushrooms, scallions, sprouts)	Wakame	Sour green apple, lemon

Some extreme yin foods that contain excess rising energy, however, can cause liver energy to rise too quickly, possibly causing migraines, and weakening the liver as toxins build up. Excess alcohol consumption, for example, can contribute to an overworked liver and can also lead to fatty liver, hepatitis, or cirrhosis. Likewise, expansive yin foods with high sugar content, such as bananas, can also weaken the liver. Although appropriate for tropical climates, these sugary foods can be too extreme for temperate climates.

Summer Energy

Ah, the fun-filled days of summer! Summer is camping outdoors, swimming in the lake, riding a bike, cooking sweet corn on the grill, and picnicking in the park. Long, warm, light-filled days abound with people sitting around the campfire, splashing in the cool water of the lake, and taking evening walks with loved ones. Like summer's abundant open blossoms, the energy is outward, expansive, and highly sustained. Summer, with the blazing hot sun at its peak, represents the fire element. The most active organ during this season is the radiant heart, with its partner the small intestine. At the height of the day, the heart peaks from 11:00 AM to 1:00 PM, and the small intestine peaks from 1:00 to 3:00 PM.

Functions of the Heart

Many energy functions vital to the health of your whole body, mind, and spirit would not be possible without the heart. The heart is the center of your body, but its capacity and power extend beyond the physical organ. A peaceful and nourished heart is the key to *wholistic* health inside and out.

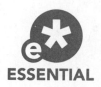

ESSENTIAL

Meditation is a *wholistic* way to balance your physical, emotional, and mental states. Studies show that meditation can improve many health conditions, reducing dependence on medications. The NIH National Center for Complementary and Alternative Medicine reports that regular meditation can reduce chronic pain, anxiety, high blood pressure, cholesterol, substance abuse, and stress hormones.

Houses Spirit

The heart is the center of your being, housing your spirit (*shen* in Chinese) on the physical plane. The best way to care for your heart for *wholistic* wellness is to listen to your inner wisdom, which is the main tool of macrobiotics. A peaceful, open heart nourished by experience and continual self-reflection manifests a balanced, full life. As the portal to your soul, the condition of the heart affects all dimensions of your body—physical, mental, emotional, and spiritual.

Governs Blood Circulation

The heart, along with the liver, governs blood circulation. Adequate blood supply and proper blood circulation nourishes normal mental activity. Also, a strong heart can supply itself with nourishing blood. Because it provides its own blood supply, it can house your spirit, which supports healthy activity in body, mind, and spirit.

Regulates Consciousness

Mental activities, such as thinking, intelligence, emotions, memory, and sleep, which fall under the umbrella of consciousness, are regulated by the heart. Mental illness and sleep abnormalities may result from an unbalanced heart. If your heart is deficient in chi, it cannot house your spirit. In this case, you may have an uneasy or restless feeling and even mental dullness and memory loss. A strong, balanced heart strengthens these important facets of consciousness.

ALERT

Harboring stress triggers many reactions that prepare the body for the "fight or flight" response. The pulse rate quickens, adrenaline surges, heart rate increases, and blood pressure rises. Habits like drinking caffeine and smoking mimic stress by increasing adrenaline production. Exposure to stress over long periods can cause inflammation and damage to blood vessels.

Governs the Tongue

The condition of the heart can be seen in the tongue. A healthy red tongue indicates balanced heart energy. However, a pale white tongue may reveal depleted heart energy, and a dark purple tongue may indicate blood stagnation. Rapid-fire speech suggests an overactive heart, whereas the inability to speak at all may indicate blockage in the heart.

Governs Blood Vessels

The state of the heart is reflected in the condition of the blood vessels, especially those in the face. A pale white complexion may indicate blood deficiency, while an overly red face may reveal excessive fire or heat. Broken blood vessels around the nose and varicose veins can also indicate hardening of the arteries.

Functions of the Small Intestine

The small intestine functions to absorb nutrients that build blood. It receives and stores partially digested food from the stomach. The small intestine then absorbs chi and water from the food and transfers residues to the large intestine for removal.

Cooking for Summer

Summer energy foods that strengthen and nourish your heart include broad leafy greens, corn, quinoa, and summer squash. Bitter taste, found in bitter greens and roasted foods, is related to summer and the fire element. Light cooking styles use a higher flame, which harmonizes with expansive summer fire energy. Summer cooking styles include:

- Blanching
- Deep-fried tempura
- Grilling
- Quick sauté with oil
- Pressed
- Raw
- Roasting

Grains	Beans	Vegetables	Sea Vegetable	Fruit
Amaranth, corn, quinoa	Kidney, lima, pinto	Broad and bitter leafy greens, string beans, radishes, summer squash	Agar, dulse, nori	Berries, watermelon

Summer growing foods are more watery and perish more quickly than those in spring. These foods, like watermelon, cucumber, and raw salads, provide the cooling effect needed to balance warm summer months. Spicy foods (garlic, ginger, and red peppers) also cool down excess body heat by bringing fire energy out, dispersing it, and then circulating it throughout the body. However, spicy foods and extremely expansive foods like sugar and chocolate can weaken already depleted heart conditions. Understanding the energetic effects of foods in your body can help you choose the appropriate foods that will balance your health condition.

Late Summer Energy

As summer winds down, late summer relaxes into lazy afternoons, football practice, and reading books on the beach. People are lying in hammocks, fruits are ripening, and high school seniors are ready to take their place as the new leaders. Late summer lasts from the beginning of August to the middle of September and corresponds to the soil element. The spleen, along with the stomach, is most active at this time of year. Soil energy is downward and settling after the intense activity of the previous season. Peak activity during the day is from 7:00 to 9:00 AM for the stomach and 9:00 to 11:00 AM for the spleen.

Functions of the Spleen

The spleen is considered to be the key organ for healthy digestion as well as several other processes in your body. In traditional Chinese medicine, the spleen is grouped together with the pancreas as a spleen system, and its functions have a closer connection to the Western pancreas. The spleen transforms and transports chi and blood, regulates water metabolism, and governs muscles, limbs, mouth, and lips.

Transforms and Transports Chi and Blood

The spleen transforms food and liquid processed by the stomach into chi and blood. The spleen also extracts nutrients from food, and then transports these nutrients all around the body. If you are always hungry, your spleen energy may be overactive from overeating, or it may be overworking because it may not be working efficiently.

Regulates Water Metabolism

The spleen also regulates water metabolism by absorbing and circulating water in the body. The spleen loathes dampness and congestion. Urinary tract infections, vaginal discharges, and candida yeast infections are conditions of depleted spleen chi. These conditions can lead to an accumulation of internal dampness, which blocks the spleen's ability to transport nourishing chi throughout the body. Signs of deficient spleen function include water retention, congestion, appetite loss, poor digestion, bloating, and weight gain.

Controls Blood Flow

One of the spleen's functions is to control blood flow in your body. Healthy spleen energy keeps the blood flowing within the blood vessels. Signs of deficient spleen function include vomiting of blood, nosebleeds, bruising, internal bleeding, and varicose veins.

FACT

Red blood cells have a life span of 120 days. Their main function is the transport of oxygen to the tissues and carbon dioxide from the lungs. Unlike most cells of the body, red blood cells do not contain a nucleus. A nucleus would take up too much space, limiting the amount of these gases a red blood cell could carry.

Governs Muscles and Limbs

Proper spleen function builds good muscle tone and warm limbs. The nutrients extracted from healthy digestion maintain muscle thickness and strength. However, atrophied muscles and cold, weak limbs indicate deficient spleen function.

Directs Ascending Chi

The spleen directs nutritive chi upward, particularly to the lung, which then distributes it to your entire body. This ascending chi holds and keeps internal organs in their place. Deficient spleen energy can cause organs to prolapse and sink. Chronic fatigue, an expression of sinking chi, can be a sign of weak spleen function.

Opens to the Mouth and Lips

Digestion begins in the mouth, and a sign of healthy spleen function is a good sense of taste. Spleen function reveals itself in the lips, which, in turn, mirror the condition of the digestive tract. When the lips are rosy pink and moist, the digestive tract is functioning well. Conversely, when the lips are pale and dry, digestion is deficient or impaired.

Houses Thought

More than one organ plays a role in regulating thought and memory. Spleen function is associated with concentration, focusing, and activities like study and memorization. Spleen chi influences your ability to perform these tasks. Deficient spleen chi manifests as cloudy thinking accompanied by a lack of concentration and poor memory. However, overthinking, extreme concentration, and overstudying can stagnate and weaken the spleen.

Functions of the Stomach

The stomach functions to receive and decompose food. It receives and stores food while partially digesting it and sending it to the small intestine. The normal function of the stomach is to direct downward movement of energy to the small intestine. Overeating and consumption of imbalanced foods creates stagnation and ascending chi, leading to acid stomach, nausea, and vomiting.

Cooking for Late Summer

As summer energy settles down, late summer plant energy reaches its peak and fruits are ripening. Foods that help strengthen the function of your spleen and stomach have downward, settling soil energy. Round vegetables that grow closer to the ground, such as onions, cabbage, and rutabagas nourish spleen energy. As the heat of summer shifts to cool, cooking styles have a warmer, settling-down energy. Cooling foods that were craved in summer, like raw salads and ice cream, put out digestive fire and deplete spleen energy. Balancing, harmonizing, centering cooking styles for late summer use a medium flame and mild seasonings. Late summer cooking styles include:

- Light stews
- Longer sauté
- Medium boil
- Nishime long steaming
- Pressed
- Quick steaming

▼ **TABLE 2-4: FOODS THAT SUPPORT SPLEEN, PANCREAS, STOMACH ENERGY**

Grains	Beans	Vegetables	Sea Vegetable	Fruit
Millet, sweet corn, sweet rice	Chickpeas, soybeans	Round vegetables (cabbage, cauliflower, onion, rutabaga, summer squash, turnip)	Arame, sea palm	Small melons, tree fruit

Sweet is the taste associated with late summer. Naturally sweet, settling foods, like sweet brown rice and millet, are balancing and support spleen function. However, concentrated sweet foods, such as refined sugar, are too extreme and can weaken digestion.

Fall Energy

Fall is the season of gathering in. Fall is raking leaves, harvesting the garden, colorful landscapes, and going back to school. Imagine pumpkins and squash, yellow mountainsides, and children waving from school bus windows. Autumn is related to the metal element, which has a downward, condensing, gathering, accumulating quality. Leaves fall off the trees and vegetation contracts as energy goes to the roots to prepare for the cold weather. The lung and its paired organ, the large intestine, are the predominant organs of fall. During the day, the lung peaks between the hours of 3:00 and 5:00 AM, and the large intestine peaks between 5:00 and 7:00 AM.

ESSENTIAL

Irritable bowel syndrome may be the gut's response to stress and emotional disturbances. Intestinal function has a strong mind-body connection. With more nerve cells in the gut than the spinal cord, the gut is considered to be the second brain. In fact, 95 percent of the body's neurotransmitter serotonin is made in the gut.

Functions of the Lung

The lung is responsible for numerous energy functions vital to your health and well-being. It controls chi, immune function, water metabolism, and blood circulation. The lung also maintains the skin, nose, and voice.

Controls Chi

The lung controls chi throughout your entire body in two ways. First, the lung governs formation of chi. The spleen, which is the major source of energy in the body, sends food chi to the lung. Once in the lung, food chi combines with air chi to form an energy that will be the basis for several other types of energy. Second, the lung distributes these several types of energy throughout the body.

Controls Immune Function

Did you know that your body has a defensive energy shield? The lung sends defensive chi (*wei chi* in Chinese) to the layer between the muscles and your skin to build up warmth and protect your body's surface. It is this reason the skin and body hair are intimately connected with the lung. Extreme environmental factors such as cold, heat, and wind can weaken your body through the skin. If your lung function is weak, your energy defense shield can become impaired, making you vulnerable to viruses. Performing breathing exercises is one way you can improve your immunity.

Maintains Skin

The lung also functions to send body fluids to the skin for moisture and nourishment. Therefore, the lung's condition is reflected in the quality of your skin. Healthy radiant skin can be an indicator of balanced lung function. However, deficient or weak lung chi can cause wrinkles along with rough, dry, or itchy skin.

Directs Descending Chi

The lung directs chi to descend in the body. If this function is blocked in some way, symptoms with ascending energy can manifest, such as asthma, phlegm, runny nose, stuffy chest, and coughing.

FACT

According to the Asthma and Allergy Foundation in America, 20 million Americans suffer from asthma. It is the most common chronic childhood disease, with nearly 5 million asthma sufferers under age 18. There are more than 4,000 deaths each year due to asthma, and 11 people die each day from this disease.

Governs Water Metabolism

The lung ensures proper water metabolism by directing water downward to be eliminated. A water imbalance can cause edema and excess phlegm in the lung. The lung and its paired organ, the large intestine, are intimately connected. If lung function is weak, the large intestine can become stagnated, and constipation or diarrhea can result as well.

Controls Blood Circulation

Proper blood circulation is dependent on healthy lung function. Although the heart controls the blood vessels, the lung creates the energy to transport the blood through them. Signs of deficient lung chi are poor blood circulation and cold hands and feet.

Opens into the Nose

In traditional Chinese medicine, the nose is the opening to the lung. When the nose is open and your sense of smell is intact, your lung function is healthy. But if your nose is stuffy and your sense of smell is lost, lung function may be imbalanced. Conversely, nosebleeds may be a sign of overheated lung chi.

Governs the Voice

Have you ever become hoarse or lost your voice with a cold? The lung is the only interior organ in direct contact with the outside world. Lung meridians run through the throat, where the larynx is located. A clear, strong, resonant voice reflects a strong lung. However, a weak lung can cause a nasal, thin, or hoarse voice, or loss of voice altogether.

Functions of the Large Intestine

The large intestine functions to absorb water from feces and eliminate waste from the body. Large intestine energy has a downward, condensing, gathering, accumulating quality that helps control rising liver energy. If large intestine energy is stagnated, however, liver energy gets stuck in the head, instead of circulating throughout the body. Signs of intestinal weakness are migraines, chronic constipation, lower abdominal pain, diarrhea, and gas. Beneficial bacteria in the intestines, which are responsible for nutrient absorption and manufacture, are destroyed by eating refined foods, stress, and antibiotics.

Cooking for Fall

Plants grown for food in autumn and winter are drier and more concentrated than those in warmer seasons. They can be kept a long time and are often stored during the cold months. Foods with pungent taste are emphasized in the fall. Foods with downward, gathering metal energy, such as root vegetables, also strengthen the lung and large intestine. Foods that support healthy intestinal function are miso and pickles that inoculate the intestines with beneficial bacteria, as well as roots and brown rice that provide downward gathering energy. Long, slow cooking, such as pressure cooking, drives energy deep into the body to strengthen your core. As late summer weather becomes cool and crisp, fall cooking becomes warmer and uses more oil and less liquid. Fall cooking styles include:

- Baking
- Broiling
- Kimpira
- Long boiling
- Long sauté
- Nishime
- Pressure cooking

▼   **TABLE 2-5: FOODS THAT SUPPORT LUNG, LARGE INTESTINE ENERGY**

Grains	Beans	Vegetables	Sea Vegetable	Fruit
Brown rice, mochi	White beans	Small contracted root vegetables (burdock, carrots, kuzu, lotus), pungent foods (daikon, watercress)	Hijiki	Hard tree fruit

Foods that can harm lung and large intestine function include cooling foods with expansive energy like spices, sugar, and alcohol. Soft, creamy foods, like ice cream, also lack gathering energy and can make the large intestine sluggish. Conversely, overly contracting foods, like baked flour products, can make the large intestine hard and inflexible. Also, mucous-causing foods, like dairy, can create congestion in the lung and large intestine.

Winter Energy

Winter means shoveling snow, cool brisk breezes, gathering friends and family together for the holidays, and preparing substantial whole grains and stews. Imagine falling snow, crackling Yule logs, fragrant herbs and seasonings, and warm sauces and soups. The element associated with winter is water, which has a floating energy. Water energy goes deep inside the earth; it is the root and basis of life. This is the time of hibernation and inward self-reflection, when the energy is still on the surface, yet active underneath.

In traditional Chinese medicine, winter is a time of conservation and storage. Because the kidney, along with the urinary bladder, is predominant in this season, winter is the time to build, conserve, and store kidney chi through rest and self-reflection. During the day, the urinary bladder peaks from 3:00 to 5:00 PM and the kidney from 5:00 to 7:00 PM.

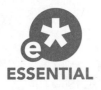

ESSENTIAL

The human body is 60 percent water. The Japanese scientist Masaru Emoto has discovered that water molecules are influenced by the energy of thoughts, words, and feelings. Since your body is composed mostly of water, his findings suggest a way to support your body's healing power through the path of intention, prayer, and gratitude.

Functions of the Kidney

The kidney performs many energy functions that are important to your overall health. The kidney is the primary source of chi for your body and helps support the function of your other organs. It also regulates water metabolism; maintains bones, teeth, and hair; and governs knees and the lower back.

Stores Kidney Essence

The kidney stores kidney essence (*jing* in Chinese), which is a combination of "inborn chi" that you inherited from your parents along with "food chi" acquired from food. Jing is then transformed into chi or blood that is used by your whole body. Inborn chi determines your mental and physical constitution as well as your life span. Inborn chi governs growth and development of your body and supports the function of your reproductive organs. Signs of deficient inborn chi can appear as infertility, impotence, and repeated miscarriages.

Regulates Water Metabolism

The kidney is responsible for water metabolism in your body. This function includes two parts. First, the kidney distributes nutritive fluid created from food chi throughout the body. Second, the kidney disposes of waste fluids that are byproducts of organ and body functions. Signs of kidney energy imbalance can manifest as edema and frequent urination. "Flushing the kidneys" by drinking excess water, as suggested by some dietary trends, can overburden and unbalance the kidney. So monitor your water intake, and drink only when you are thirsty.

Maintains Bones and Teeth

The kidney nourishes the skeletal system, bone marrow, brain, and spinal cord. Osteoporosis can reflect disrupted energy at a deep level as well as overall body weakness. The teeth are considered to be extensions of the bone and are also supported by kidney chi. Tooth decay at an early age can also indicate weak kidney function.

Governs the Knees

Healthy kidney function manifests as strong, supple knees. Kidney chi naturally declines with age, so it is common for your knees to become weaker as you grow older.

Opens into the Ears

The ears are the opening of the kidney. Earaches, tinnitus, excess ear-wax, and loss of hearing can indicate deficient kidney chi.

FACT

Maintaining Head Hair

Kidney essence (jing) changes into chi and blood. Blood nourishes your hair, so healthy hair is a sign of balanced kidney function. However, hair loss, graying, and brittle hair can indicate kidney energy deficiency.

Controls the Lower Back

The kidneys themselves are located in the lower back area, so this part of the body is associated with kidney chi. Foods that weaken kidney chi, such as meat, coffee, and soymilk, can also create chronic low back pain.

Functions of the Urinary Bladder

The urinary bladder functions to receive, store, and excrete urine from the body. Urine is made by the filtering process of the kidney. Urinary bladder function is controlled by kidney chi. All urinary problems result from deficient kidney and urinary bladder functions.

Cooking for Winter

Foods with floating water energy go deep into the body and strengthen the kidney, urinary bladder, and reproductive organs. So the most beneficial foods for this time of year are deeply strengthening burdock, buckwheat, black soybeans, and black sesame seeds. Dried foods, like dried mushrooms, also contain concentrated energy to build inner strength. The taste associated with winter and the water element is salty, so sea vegetables are strengthening to the kidney. Winter cooking includes warming soups, more oil, less liquid, fish, and rich bean dishes. Cooking styles that incorporate warming energy into the food include:

- Baking
- Deep frying
- Dehydrating
- Long boiling
- Long picking
- Pressure cooking
- Pressed
- Stews
- Multiple combination cooking

▼ **TABLE 2-6: FOODS THAT SUPPORT KIDNEY, BLADDER ENERGY**

Grains	Beans	Vegetables	Sea Vegetable	Fruit
Buckwheat	Aduki, black soybeans	Root plants, dried roots	Kombu	Dried or storable tree fruit

Multiple combination cooking means using many cooking styles in one dish, as in fried rice, in which rice is first boiled and then fried. Adding multiple cooking styles to a dish increases its warming energy, which strengthens your body deep inside. In contrast, foods that can harm kidney function are cooling foods, like salads, tropical fruits, and sugar.

CHAPTER 3

The Kitchen as Macrobiotic Playground

Remember how your mom used to tell you not to play with your food? Well, now you can. Think of the kitchen as a macrobiotic playground, an opportunity to play in the sandbox and learn how energy of seasons, food, and cooking techniques contribute to achieving a healthy balanced lifestyle. You connect with the essence of cooking by expanding your perceptions and tapping into intuition and creativity. Before playing with your food, set the intention to be open to inspiration and to have fun.

Tapping into Intuition

For many people, the very term macrobiotic is intimidating and challenges today's lifestyle of busy schedules, e-mail conversations, and fast food. In a back-to-nature way of living, life slows down, and you become inspired to develop not only recipes, but also a deeper connection with inner awareness and a gratitude for life. As you develop an intimate relationship with food, you learn to listen to intuition and trust it to guide you back to your center. Using food as a path to wholeness can help you become empowered to bring about inner and outer healing, while simultaneously moving from chaos back to harmony.

ESSENTIAL

Intuition is a valuable self-development tool that you can use to bring balance into your life. Intuition can help you tune into life and confirm you are on your path. Intuitive messages may alert you to possible danger. You can also develop a more intimate connection and increased trust in your higher power.

Focusing on intellectual development, while neglecting creativity, is one-sided. Tapping into intuition through macrobiotic cooking can help you develop a more *wholistic* awareness.

Building a New Recipe

Following a recipe to the letter can be a learning experience for those new to macrobiotic cooking. However, if you prefer to exercise your freedom and creativity and enjoy a variety of meals, you can create brand new recipes or alter current recipes to make them your own. Creating new recipes may seem overwhelming at first, but the basic concepts are simple and you can apply them whenever you cook to make many new creations.

Main Ingredients

Main ingredients make up the majority of the dish and set the direction for the recipe. They may be grains, beans, or vegetables or a combination of each. Since main ingredients may have different cooking times, the cooking method may be different for each ingredient as well. If so, ingredients may be added to a dish at separate intervals to avoid overcooking or undercooking. Or, ingredients may be cooked separately prior to mixing them together at the end.

QUESTION

Does cooking food destroy enzymes?
There is a question as to whether the enzymes in raw food are needed for digestion. Plant enzymes are used for plant growth and decomposition after harvesting. Cooking destroys these plant enzymes, but these plant enzymes are not used for human digestion anyway. Humans secrete their own digestive enzymes from glands in the digestive system.

Cooking Methods

Besides providing important nutrients, such as protein, carbohydrates, vitamins, and minerals for healthy organ and immune functions, the role of food in health is important in maintaining overall energetic balance of the body. Eating seasonal food imbued with life energy can nourish your body from the inside out. Adjusting the cooking styles to balance your constitution and condition can help you prevent and recover from illness as well.

▼ TABLE 3-1: LONG-, MEDIUM-, AND SHORT-COOKED DISHES

Long Cooked	Medium Cooked	Short Cooked
Beans, grains, kimpira, long fermented pickles, nishime, pressure cooked sea vegetable dishes, soups, stews	Boiled, sautéed, steamed, stir fry	Blanched vegetables, steamed greens, quick sautés, quick steamed, pressed salad, quick pickles, raw salad

The method of cooking is important in balancing the energy of the dish with the seasons. Long-cooked foods are more appropriate in cool weather, while short-cooked foods are more appealing in warm weather. In summer, a refreshing Hazelnut Amasake Kanten Parfait with Berry Good Jam (page 202) cools you down, whereas in winter, a steaming bowl of delicious homemade Turkish Lentil Soup (page 172) warms you from head to toe. To support your organs and for dynamic energy, include a variety of long- or medium-cooked and short-cooked dishes on the plate.

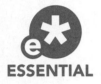

ESSENTIAL

Fresh-picked and raw vegetables usually have the highest nutritional content. However, some phytochemicals are bio-available only after the vegetables are cooked. For example, cooked carrots are better sources of an antioxidant called beta-carotene than raw carrots. Variety in cooking methods as well as in vegetables is the key to obtaining the widest possible array of phytochemicals.

Balancing Flavors in a Recipe

While ingredients are cooking, flavors may be enhanced or balanced using the highest quality organic seasonings available. Avoid or reduce all commercial seasonings and all hot spices or stimulating herbs, as they can have extreme effects on health. The five main tastes in macrobiotic cooking are sour, bitter, sweet, pungent, and salty. When you balance flavors in a recipe, you will most often use sources of sweet, sour, or salty tastes. Pungent and bitter tastes are optional, depending on the dish. Refer to Appendix C for a list of seasonings and sources of five tastes to keep on hand.

Sources of Sweet Taste

Sweet flavor supports the spleen, pancreas, and stomach organs, and usually comes from complex carbohydrates in sweet vegetables, such as butternut squash and cabbage, and whole grains. Even plain brown rice becomes sweet when chewed, as the amylase enzyme in saliva changes complex carbohydrates into simple sugars. Sweet flavor provides relaxing energy to balance the contracting energy of salt. A mild sweet taste should predominate your meals, with sour, salty, bitter, and pungent tastes used as accents throughout the day. In a meal, the ratio of sweet to other tastes is approximately 75 percent mild sweet taste to 5–7 percent of each of the others in Table 3-2.

Salt Sources

The most common seasoning is sea salt and other salt sources, such as miso, shoyu, and tamari. Add salt sources during cooking rather than at the table to allow salt to be absorbed into the food for more balanced energy. Unrefined sea salt that is stone ground and has balanced minerals is best, but avoid Celtic Grey sea salt, which is highly concentrated in minerals, and therefore, very contracting.

Table salt usually comes from salt mines and is refined to remove most minerals until it is pure sodium chloride. Studies have linked table salts to hypertension and other heart or blood illness. Sea salt, however, is unrefined salt derived directly from a living ocean or sea and contains about 80 mineral elements that the body needs.

Miso and shoyu that is fermented for 2–3 years contain healthful living enzymes and beneficial organisms like lactobacillus. Tamari, which is a by-product of making miso, is used minimally as it has a heavier, more contracting energy compared to miso or shoyu. However, use all salt sources in moderate, balanced amounts for light taste and improved health, as over use of salt may lead to sweet cravings.

Sources of Sour Taste

Sour flavor, which balances liver and gallbladder energy, appears in sauerkraut or lemon juice in dressings. The upward energy of sour seasonings is important to balance contracting energy of salt. Sour flavor can act as an accent, such as a splash of lemon juice that brings brightness and pizzazz to a dish. Or sour flavor can be a main component, helping to showcase a dish, such as Lemon Millet Bars (page 208).

Sources of Bitter Taste

Include bitter flavors to nourish the heart and small intestine, using bitter greens, such as kale or dandelion greens. One way to add bitter taste to a recipe is to use parsley as a garnish. Or you can add chopped greens to soup at the end of cooking. Roasted nuts can also add bitter flavor as well as crunch to a recipe.

Sources of Pungent Taste

Pungent foods, such as grated daikon or mustard, disperse and move congestion in the lung and large intestine. Garnish a dish with raw chopped scallions or chives to add pungent taste. Or use ginger during cooking to incorporate pungent flavor into your recipe.

▼ TABLE 3-2: TASTES FOR BUILDING A NEW RECIPE

Taste	Supported Organs	Sources of Taste
Sweet	Spleen, pancreas, stomach	Amasake, apple juice, barley malt syrup, brown rice syrup, chestnuts, mirin, sweet vegetables, whole grains
Salt	Kidney, bladder	Miso, sauerkraut, sea salt, shiso leaves, shoyu, tamari, tekka, umeboshi plum, umeboshi vinegar
Sour	Liver, gallbladder	Brown rice vinegar, lemon, lime, mustard, orange, sauerkraut juice, shiso leaves, umeboshi plum, umeboshi vinegar
Bitter	Heart, small intestine	Broad leafy greens (kale), cilantro, grain coffee, parsley, roasted nuts and seeds
Pungent	Lung, large intestine	Garlic, ginger, horseradish, leek, mild spices, mustard, onion, raw leafy greens (watercress), scallion, shallot

Each ingredient has an important role not only in building recipes but also in contributing to your overall health. Not all recipes have all five tastes. However, include all five tastes on the plate to activate all areas of the palate and balance the energy of the body organs.

Using Herbs

A grain- and vegetable-based diet becomes more tasteful with the use of fresh and dried herbs and spices, which add flavor and nutrition as well as enhance digestion. Based on traditional dietary practices around the world, particular herbs and spices in a dish identify its international flavor. Cilantro is associated with Mexican dishes, oregano with Italian, marjoram with French, and ginger with Chinese. Mild herbs, which are leaves of low growing shrubs, are an easy way to enhance a dish and infuse flavor into oils, marinades, and sauces. The most common herbs to use are:

- Basil
- Caraway
- Cilantro
- Dill
- Oregano
- Parsley
- Rosemary
- Sage
- Tarragon
- Thyme

QUESTION

Are cilantro and coriander interchangeable in recipes?
Both cilantro and coriander come from the same plant, known as cilantro plant. However, their flavors are very different and cannot be substituted for each other. Cilantro refers to the wide delicate lacy green leaves with a pungent flavor, while coriander is a spice made from the seed of the cilantro plant.

Dried herbs, which are more pungent and concentrated than fresh, can be added during cooking. However, to preserve flavor and aroma, add fresh herbs toward the end of cooking. To substitute fresh herbs in place of dried, use the following equivalents: 1 tablespoon finely sliced fresh herbs = 1 teaspoon crumpled dried herbs or ¼–½ teaspoon ground dried herbs.

Spices originate from the bark, root, seed, berry, bud, or fruit of tropical plants and trees. Curries and other hot spices harmonize best with hot weather and are often used in tropical climates to promote perspiration to cool the body. Used minimally, herbs and spices can retain the flavor of food, while eliminating or reducing the need for fat, sugar, or salt. Sweet-tasting spices used for desserts or to reduce sugar cravings include:

- Allspice
- Anise
- Cardamom
- Cinnamon
- Cloves
- Ginger
- Mace
- Nutmeg

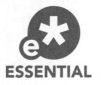

ESSENTIAL

Taste and smell your herbs and spices before you add them to a recipe. These two senses are intimately connected and can help you become more familiar with signature flavors and aromas. You will not only develop an intuitive sense for which herbs and spices to use, you will learn to trust yourself to make substitutions.

Spices and dried herbs can also add a warming energy and meaty flavor to dishes. Some warming spices, like cinnamon and ginger, counteract the cooling effect of fruit and vegetables. For example, a few red pepper flakes can lighten and energize the heavy, dense energy of tempeh or seitan, transforming them into meatier, more digestible foods. This balancing of light herbs and spices with heavy and bland foods is the epitome of the art of macrobiotic cooking. Yet, there are some side effects of overusing herbs and spices. Some spices like curry and chili powder, for instance, can be irritating to the gastrointestinal tract. Although certain fresh herbs, like basil and fresh hot peppers, help disperse the heavy quality and excess heat of meats, poultry, and cheeses, these herbs can also be weakening for vegans.

FACT

Once considered in Egypt to be more valuable than gold, cinnamon is one of the oldest known spices and medicines. Its health benefits come from the essential oils that are antimicrobial, anti-inflammatory, and anti-clotting. Studies also show that including cinnamon in the diet reduces the risk factors associated with diabetes and cardiovascular diseases.

Ways to Amp Up Flavor

Imagine your meals so appealing and appetizing they make your mouth water to think of them. Using seasonings such as herbs and spices is one way to amp up flavor for the mainstay dishes of the grain, bean, vegetables, and greens. Additional ways to amp up flavor and turn ordinary ingredients into a decadent gourmet experience are sauces, color, texture, and creativity itself.

Sauces

Luscious, tantalizing sauces are the soul of macrobiotic cooking, bringing life to a plate of otherwise ordinary food. They can make or break a dish, transforming an everyday meal into gourmet cuisine. Colorful red, green, and yellow sauces enliven the plate—as well as the palate—and make mealtimes fun and inspiring. Unlike traditional sauces and gravies that use fat, white flour, and artificial chemicals, macrobiotic sauces use healthy and energetically balanced ingredients that provide flavor and nourish the body. Sauces are also a great way to get children and reluctant adults to eat their bitter greens.

Macrobiotic sauces contain four basic components: base, liquid, salt, and sour taste. The base is the thickener for the sauce that is then thinned with liquid. The liquid is drizzled slowly into the base until the desired consistency is reached. Examples of liquids are vegetable or sea vegetable stock, juice, vegan milk, vinegar, mirin, water, and oil. Depending on the sauce, the salt and sour taste may be optional. Aromatic seasonings, such as herbs, add another layer of flavor to the sauce. By experimenting with the amounts and flavors of different ingredients, you can transform a recipe to create a new sensation. There are four basic macrobiotic sauces: reduction sauces, vegetable-based sauces, gravies, and nut- or seed-based sauces.

Reduction Sauces

Reduction sauces are seasoned liquids that are reduced over low heat until the flavors are concentrated into thick syrup. These sauces are used as glazes or to garnish a dish. You can make a simple reduction sauce with balsamic vinegar that is simmered over low heat until it thickens. You can even make a teriyaki soy sauce to create a teriyaki glaze for tempeh, by reducing apple juice, brown rice vinegar, and tamari soy sauce. Delicious syrup for poached pears is easy to make by reducing apple juice, maple syrup, cloves, star anise, and orange rind.

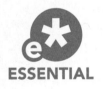

ESSENTIAL

A member of the legume family, kuzu is prized in China and Japan for its medicinal uses for relieving diarrhea, over-acidity, bacterial infection, and alcohol cravings. Kuzu also contains a high concentration of flavonoids, which are beneficial for alleviating migraines, lowering cholesterol, reducing the formation of blood clots, and preventing heart disease.

Vegetable-Based Sauces

Vegetable-based sauces use puréed beans, vegetables, tofu, or cooked grains as the base, which is thinned with a little water. First steam, sauté, simmer, or pressure cook colorful vegetables in a small amount of water until soft. Then blend them or put through a food mill with seasonings such as herbs, umeboshi paste, miso, or shoyu.

Gravies

Gravies are clear sauces thickened with kuzu, arrowroot, or whole grain flour dissolved in cold water. Kuzu helps strengthen the intestines and is used to balance nausea by focusing energy downward in the abdomen. To use kuzu, the kuzu-water mixture must be added to a heated sauce at the end of cooking and then simmered for a couple of minutes to thicken. You can make simple gravies using sautéed onions, water, tamari, and kuzu.

Besides thickening gravies and vegetable dishes, kuzu and arrowroot can make desserts and puddings creamy. Kuzu is also used with agar to solidify fruit or amasake desserts, such as kantens and pies. Another function of arrowroot is to take the place of eggs to thicken desserts. To replace one egg, use 2 tablespoons arrowroot flour.

Nut- or Seed-Based Sauces

Nut- or seed-based sauces use nuts, seeds, nut butters, or seed butters and generally need no thickener or reduction. Some nut- or seed based sauces are not cooked, but—like Basil Pine Nut Pesto (page 182)—are just puréed in a blender or suribachi bowl. Some tahini and nut butters are heated together with umeboshi or tamari soy sauce and water to make a simple but tasty sauce. Nut and seed butters also contain oil, so it may not be necessary to add more oil. You can make an easy dressing by grinding roasted pumpkin seeds with water, umeboshi paste, and scallions.

Color

Look to nature for inspiration in designing your meals. Imagine that your plate is the canvas and your foods are the pigments you will use to create your nutritional masterpiece. Paint your canvas with the colorful pigments in your food. Using at least three colors on the plate maximizes visual interest as well as ensures a variety of nutritious vegetables. A plate of dilled beet pickles, kidney bean chili, and red wehani rice is monochromatic and overwhelming with one defined color. However, serving marinated green beans, roasted butternut squash, and brown rice croquettes distributes various colors throughout the plate, breaks up the monotony, and adds dynamic energy.

Texture

Even serving delicious puréed foods at every meal can get boring after a while. Like color, a variety of textures adds dynamic energy and contrast, which makes meals more interesting. Healthy crunchy, chewy, and creamy foods provide texture to enliven an otherwise dull plate. Refer to Table 3-3 for ways to add texture to meals.

FACT

The more colors on the plate, the more health-promoting properties there are as well. The colors in vegetables give hints about their vitamin content. Dark leafy greens are high in B vitamins, while red and yellow vegetables are good sources of vitamins A and C. Eating a wide variety of different colored vegetables ensures a broad spectrum of essential vitamins.

▼   **TABLE 3-3: WAYS TO ADD TEXTURE**

Crunch	Chewy	Creamy
Roasted sea vegetables, gomashio, roasted nuts and seeds, crisp vegetables, pressed salads, quick pickled vegetables	Grains, noodles, mochi, tempeh	Sauces, nut and seed butters, puréed soups, porridges, well-cooked beans

Creativity

Food that is visually appealing attracts the senses and nourishes the soul. When the plate looks appetizing, it probably is, and you can feel life energy emanating from it. Possible ideas for your canvas plate include:

- Use a variety of vegetables and cut them into matchsticks, rounds, half-moons, or cubes to add visual interest.

- Food that is wrapped in nori sheets or tortillas is perfect for fast food or travel meals.
- Get in touch with your inner child. Form seasoned cooked grains into shapes and sprinkle roasted nuts on top.

Gourmet chefs know that visually appealing dishes sell themselves. Food plating is a required course at chef schools, where students learn how to balance every aspect of cooking. You can learn about the Zen art of balance in your own kitchen using your intuition, which is your wisest guide.

Substituting Ingredients

As you begin building recipes, you may find that some ingredients are unavailable or allergies may prevent their use. Or you may want to replace high-fat ingredients with ones that are low-fat and more energetically balanced. Substitutions that work introduce new ingredients, while keeping the basic essence and flavor of a dish. The following are some examples of substitutions:

- Tempeh, mushrooms, seitan, or burdock can take the place of meat in vegetarian gravies, beans, and sautés.
- Exchange mushrooms in a dish with nuts, tempeh, or burdock to create new versions.
- Grated mochi stirred into a hot dish can mimic the consistency of cheese.
- Puréeing soups or adding vegan milk or tahini creates creamy texture in place of dairy.
- Add umeboshi paste to sauces or soups to create a flavor similar to that of tomato.
- Smoked dulse mimics the flavor and texture of bacon and can be added to salads, fried rice, and sandwiches.

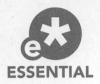

Food allergies can be related to intestinal problems, such as leaky gut syndrome. As large protein molecules enter abnormally large spaces in the intestinal wall, an allergic reaction occurs as antibodies to these proteins enter the blood. Crohn's disease is another intestinal disorder related to food allergies, because small intestine inflammation causes sensitivity to certain foods.

▼ TABLE 3-4: SUGGESTIONS FOR VEGETABLE SUBSTITUTIONS

Vegetable	Substitution
Fresh beans	Green beans, edamame, fava beans, peas, snow peas, sugar snap peas, wax beans
Fennel	Anise, caraway, licorice
Alliums	Chives, leeks, onions, scallions, shallots
Potato	Celery root, Jerusalem artichoke (sunchoke), rutabaga, sweet potato
Summer squash	Crookneck squash, patty pan squash, yellow squash, zucchini
Sweet vegetables	Beet, cabbage, carrot, corn, onion, parsnip, winter squash, yam

Go to farmers' markets and become familiar with the locally grown, seasonal organic foods, which are energetically balanced with the natural environment. Develop a relationship with your food by focusing on one vegetable to use each week. Think of innovative ways to incorporate your featured vegetable into various dishes and new recipes. You'll not only become more intimate with your weekly vegetable, but you'll also deepen your intuition and connection with nature.

CHAPTER 4

Menu Planning

If you are new to macrobiotics, you may feel overwhelmed about creating new recipes and shopping for new ingredients. A menu plan you can incorporate into your busy life uses helpful tools to simplify the process. With the right tools, you can choose menu plans that fulfill dietary needs, get recipes, and even use a shopping list to lessen stress or help with ailments or weakness. The small steps you take now will lead to giant leaps later as you develop confidence to create something new and feel inspired to develop your practice further.

Developing Meals

Just as restaurants have soup of the day (soup du jour), featuring the chef's special creation, you can designate a one-of-kind dish for each day of the week. Create your favorite meal for each day of the week and design a menu around that. This will establish a natural rhythm that helps you harmonize your meals with new recipes. Find possible meal-of-the-day ideas in Table 4-1.

▼ **TABLE 4-1: MEAL-OF-THE-DAY IDEAS**

Day	Meal
Sunday	Vegetarian pizza
Monday	Quick meal: burrito, sushi, etc.
Tuesday	Pasta: udon, vegetable, and bean salad
Wednesday	Pressure cooked rice, chickpeas, and kale
Thursday	Vegetable casserole
Friday	Bean soup with rice and two vegetables
Saturday	Stir-fried rice or noodles with vegetables

Developing menu plans is a process of learning to do things differently from your regular routine. Table 4-2 is a blank weekly menu plan; underlined grain and bean means they need to be soaked. Use a clipboard with the week's menu to add recipes, and note which ingredients to buy on a shopping list. Underline or include a list of ingredients to soak for the next day's dinner. Refer to Appendix A for ready-made, seasonal menu plans. Encourage your creative juices to flow by adding a new recipe a week. As you become more comfortable creating menu plans and recipes, eventually, your intuition will be your guide.

Weekday	Breakfast	Lunch	Snack	Dinner
Meal Components	Grain porridge; Vegetables; Condiment; Beverage	Grain; Bean; Vegetable; Soup; Pickle; Condiment; Beverage	Snack	Grain; Bean or fish; Vegetable; Greens; Sea vegetable; Pickle; Condiment; Beverage; Dessert (optional)
SUNDAY				
MONDAY				
TUESDAY				
WEDNESDAY				
THURSDAY				
FRIDAY				
SATURDAY				

Dinner

Imagine coming home after work and finding a delicious, organic, macrobiotic dinner prepared just for you. As your own chef, you can prepare the most luscious and tantalizing nutritious meals that your palate could ever imagine. Design your menu plan around dinner, because it is usually the largest and most elaborate meal of the day. Simplify dinner into three components: grain, protein, and vegetable.

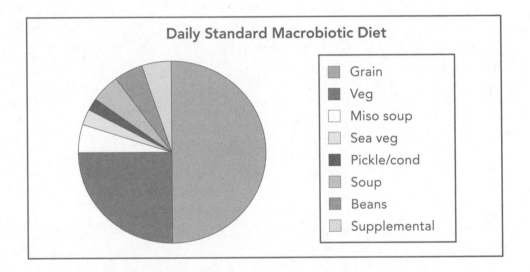

▼ TABLE 4-3: DAILY STANDARD MACROBIOTIC DIET

Food	Amount
Whole grains or grain products	50–60 percent by weight
Vegetables	25–30 percent by weight
Beans or Fish	5–10 percent by weight
Soup	5–10 percent by weight
Sea vegetables	2–5 percent by weight
Supplemental foods: Fruit, desserts, beverages, condiments, seasonings, snacks, garnishes	Small amounts of each

Grains

A healing diet uses whole grains to help maintain blood sugar levels, since intact whole grain fiber slows down the absorption of sugar into the blood. In this diet, 50–60 percent by weight (or ⅓ by volume) of your daily total intake is whole grain, and some grain is included at each meal. Pressure cook or boil whole grains in a heavy pot with a heavy lid, such as cast-iron enameled cookware. A great option is to use a ceramic or glass Ohsawa pot inside the pressure cooker, which makes the rice softer and richer tasting than boiling or pressure cooking alone. Cook grain with a stamp-sized piece of kombu per 1 cup of whole grain or with ⅛ teaspoon sea salt per cup of grain. Water to grain ratio is 1 part whole grains to 1–1½ parts water. The staple grain is brown rice, which has complete balanced carbohydrates, fats, proteins, and minerals. Eat whole grain brown rice daily and use leftovers within 24–48 hours. Secondary whole grains can be mixed with brown rice or eaten separately.

▼ TABLE 4-4: RELATIONSHIP OF WHOLE GRAINS AND SUPPORTED ORGANS

Supported Organs	Whole Grain	Cracked Grain
Liver, gallbladder	Barley, wheat, rye, whole oats	Bulgur, couscous, rolled oats, steel cut oats, flour
Heart, small intestine	Corn, quinoa, amaranth	Corn grits, flour
Spleen, pancreas, stomach	Millet	Flour, millet grits
Lung, large intestine	Brown rice	Flour, brown rice grits
Kidney, bladder	Buckwheat	Flour, buckwheat grits

Cracked (refined) grains and flour products, such as noodles and bread, may also be used occasionally, depending on health condition. Experiment with various brown rice–secondary grain combinations and brown rice–bean combinations. By cooking grains and beans together, you can save time by creating one dish instead of two.

Protein

Beans are high in protein and should make up 5–10 percent by weight of your total daily food intake (½–1 cup beans per day). Except for soft, light beans such as lentils and split peas, most beans are hard and need to be soaked overnight to improve digestibility. To remove gas, throw away soaking water, except when soaking aduki beans and black soybeans from Hokkaido, Japan, as this water is medicinal. Cook aduki beans and black soybeans in this soaking water.

FACT

Aduki beans grown in the volcanic soil of northern island of Hokkaido, Japan, have a high mineral content and are lower in fat and oil than any other bean. With a shinier surface and deeper maroon color, Hokkaido adukis can be distinguished from North American adukis, which have a dull surface and lighter red color.

To cook beans, bring them to a boil and skim off the gas-causing foam that rises to the top. If you are cooking a brown rice–bean combo, boil beans separately, remove foam, add the rice, and continue to cook. Always cook beans with a stamp-sized piece of kombu (or bay leaf) to add minerals and soften the beans, making a more balanced digestible dish. Season beans at the end when they are 80 percent done with salt or soy sauce (¼–½ teaspoon per cup per day) or add miso. When pressure cooking, cook beans until done, season the beans, and cook another 5 minutes uncovered. Eat beans every day (½ cup each for lunch and dinner), except on the days when you are having fish or another protein source. To retain nutrients, use up bean dishes within 1–2 days.

▼ **TABLE 4-5: RELATIONSHIP OF BEANS AND SUPPORTED ORGANS**

Supported Organs	Bean
Liver, gallbladder	Edamame, lentil, peas
Heart, small intestine	Kidney, pinto

Supported Organs	Bean
Spleen, pancreas, stomach	Chickpea (garbanzo)
Lung, large intestine	White beans (great northern, navy)
Kidney, bladder	Aduki, black soybean

Fish is an easily digested protein that is an alternative to beans. Eat non-fatty white meat fish (sole, trout, carp, halibut, flounder, red snapper, haddock, cod, and scrod) 1–3 times a week, depending on your health. Fatty fish is high in omega-3 fatty acids, which are essential acids important in maintaining cardiovascular and brain function. Red meat fish (salmon, tuna, etc.), shellfish (shrimp, crab, clams, etc.), and blue-skinned fish (herring, sardines, etc.) are an occasional-use fatty fish as they contain excess contracting energy. Recommended cooking styles are steaming, poaching, boiling, or cooked in soup. Contracting cooking styles—broiling, grilling, baking, smoking, and deep frying—are used occasionally. A portion size is 4–6 ounces, about the size of a deck of cards. Serve fish with grated raw daikon, grated radish, grated ginger, lemon, or grated horseradish to help dissolve fats in the fish. Serve with plenty of vegetables and leafy greens to balance the contracting energy of fish.

Vegetables

About 25–30 percent of the weight of your total daily food intake should be bright, vibrant vegetables that enliven a plate with color and flavor. To add dynamic energy and support various organs, vary both the cooking styles (soups, water or oil sautéed, steamed, or stewed) and the type of vegetables used each day. Short-cooked vegetable dishes, like steamed broccoli or blanched kale, are best made before each meal. Long-cooked vegetable dishes, like carrot and burdock kimpira, are best eaten within 24 hours, and may be reheated and eaten as leftovers the next day. Make a crispy dish of at least one leafy green daily. Steam or blanch greens until soft and just turning bright green, but avoid overcooking.

Supported Organs	Vegetables
Liver, gallbladder	Young leafy greens (baby bok choy, spring greens) and upward growing plants (celery, chives, leeks, mushrooms, scallions, sprouts)
Heart, small intestine	Bitter and broad leafy greens (arugula, carrot tops, collards, dandelion greens, daikon tops, kale, radish tops, turnip tops)
Spleen, pancreas, stomach	Round vegetables (cabbage, cauliflower, onion, rutabaga, winter squash)
Lung, large intestine	Root vegetables (burdock, carrot, daikon, lotus root, parsnip, radish)
Kidney, bladder	Dried vegetables (dried daikon, dried shiitake, dried lotus root) and root vegetables

Lunch

Lunch can be as elaborate as fresh grains, protein, and vegetables served with soup, or as simple as leftovers from dinner from the night before. Depending on your schedule, you can choose to combine breakfast and lunch for a combo brunch or make it a separate meal. Time-saving steps also help streamline the process of making lunch. Refer to Table 4-7 for quick meal ideas.

▼ TABLE 4-7: QUICK 10–15 MINUTE MEALS

Meal	Preparation
Burgers	Make grain or bean burgers ahead of time and keep in refrigerator ready to fry and serve with pre-made mushroom gravy.
Corn on the cob	Boil corn on the cob for 10 minutes and serve with umeboshi paste, or cut off cooked corn kernels to mix with vegetables and salads.

Meal	Preparation
Grains	Choose quick-cooking grains like couscous, quinoa, or bulgur, add sautéed vegetables, and serve with a tasty sauce.
Noodles	Cook noodles with green onion and vegetables.
Mochi	Fry mochi or polenta squares in sesame oil and serve with bean salad and greens.
Sandwich	Make tempeh sandwiches with pre-cooked tempeh, sauerkraut, mustard, and sourdough bread, and fill with sprouts, lettuce, and pumpkin seed spread. (Natural [un-yeasted] sourdough is preferred to commercial yeasted breads that are too expanded [yin] and ungrounded for the intestines.)
Sauces	Delicious dressings and sauces made ahead of time spruce up quick burritos or salads.
Spreads	Make hummus and spread on sourdough bread, crackers, or rice cakes.
Soup	Make soup and add leftover beans and grains, or add rice noodles to miso soup with matchstick carrots.
Taco	Reheat beans and add them to a crispy pan-fried tortilla shell with lettuce and pre-made cilantro onion dressing.

Breakfast

Beginning the day with a balanced meal gives you strength and energy that sustains you. Breakfast usually consists of cooked whole grains and water made into rich creamy porridge, with or without vegetables. You can use leftover grains from dinner for a quick porridge that takes just 10 minutes. Sweeten plain porridge with amasake, brown rice syrup, or jam made with sweet vegetables or fruit. Serve bright green leafy vegetables as a side dish to balance the heavier grains. Miso soup cooked with wakame and vegetables is optional. (Because miso soup activates digestion, you may feel hungry throughout the day if you eat miso soup for breakfast.)

Supplement Dishes

Limiting the complexity of your meals is the first step to incorporating macrobiotics into your busy life. Developing menu plans helps you bridge recipes, meals, and shopping list into a seamless process. It is helpful to start with the basic meals of dinner, lunch, and breakfast, and then fill in the gaps with additional smaller dishes when you feel comfortable. When you are ready, you can supplement your menu plan with sea vegetables, soups, condiments, pickles, beverages, desserts, and snacks.

Sea Vegetables

Mother Nature, in her cosmic wisdom, has demonstrated her marvelous skill in cultivating nutritious sea vegetables, which contain all the essentials of life to provide strength, vitality, vigor, and energy. Marine biologists and ecologists have recognized that sea vegetables have the ability to take up minerals from the water and hold onto these minerals in their cells. This ability makes organic sea vegetables a rich source of eighty essential minerals, including magnesium, calcium, iron, and iodine. Supporting the kidney and reproductive organs, sea vegetables are eaten daily in the form of a ½ sheet of nori or another sea vegetable cooked in a vegetable dish. To flavor broths, use wakame or kombu, both of which contain glutamine, a natural monosodium glutamate. Besides softening beans, kombu has the ability to soften tumors and masses and should not be eaten excessively during pregnancy. Refer to Table 4-8 for the most commonly used sea vegetables and their descriptions. Other sea vegetables, such as agar (used for vegetable dishes, aspics, desserts), dulse, Irish moss, mekabu, and sea palm are optional.

▼ **TABLE 4-8: MOST COMMONLY USED SEA VEGETABLES**

Sea Vegetable	How Often to Use	Description
Nori	½ sheet daily	Dark, purple black sheets; sushi nori reduces blood cholesterol, functions as anti-blood coagulant, and is antitumor.
Wakame	Daily in soup	Long, wavy strips; reduces breast cancer, promotes weight loss, and lowers cholesterol.

Sea Vegetable	How Often to Use	Description
Kombu	Daily in beans and grains	Thick, dark, strips; reduces blood cholesterol and hypertension.
Arame	Either arame or hijiki ⅓–⅔ cup 2–3 times a week	Lacy, wiry sea vegetable; milder in flavor compared to hijiki and is anticancer.
Hijiki	Either arame or hijiki ⅓–⅔ cup 2–3 times a week	Resembles black wiry hair; high in calcium and potassium and strengthens bones, teeth, hair, and nails.

ESSENTIAL

Deeply growing hijiki, kombu, arame, and agar all carry downward energy to help in recovery from chemotherapy and radiation, which go deep into the body. These sea vegetables are deeply strengthening miracle workers that help discharge toxins by binding heavy metals and radioactive substances and purging them downward and out of the body.

Soups

About 5–10 percent by weight of the total daily food consumption should include soup. A steaming bowl of soup eaten at the beginning of a meal prepares the stomach to receive food and stimulates digestive secretions. Eat one bowl of miso soup almost daily. Miso soup provides lactobacillus bacteria to help recover intestinal flora, especially after sugar consumption. To preserve beneficial bacteria, add miso (1 teaspoon per cup of liquid) at the end of cooking, and never boil miso soup. Like wine, miso comes in many varieties and flavors, including barley, aduki, chickpea, brown rice, and sweet white miso. Always cook miso soup with a small amount of wakame (¼"–½" piece per cup of soup), and vary the type of vegetables used daily. Occasionally, add dried shiitake mushrooms, soaked and finely chopped. Add leafy greens toward the end of cooking, to retain their green color and preserve freshness.

In addition to miso soup, make another kind of soup often during the week. Season your soup in moderation with miso, soy sauce, or sea salt, using ¼–½ teaspoon seasoning per 4 cups water. To add freshness, garnish with finely chopped parsley or scallions. Soup that is cooked longer may be served a second time as leftovers the next day.

ALERT

Vitamin B12, produced by intestinal bacteria, is a water-soluble vitamin necessary for proper brain and nerve function, blood formation, and DNA synthesis. Animal products and supplements are the most reliable sources of vitamin B12, as miso, storebought tempeh, and sea vegetables contain an analogue that is biologically inactive.

Condiments

In addition to seasoning a grain or vegetable dish, condiments are useful for balancing the meal, aiding digestion, and alkalinizing the blood. A variety of condiments are kept on the table and used moderately according to each individual's taste and health condition. Main condiments that should always be on the table include:

- Gomashio
- Umeboshi plums
- Shiso leaves powder
- Tekka
- Sea vegetable powder
- Green nori flakes (ao nori sea vegetable)

Sprinkle sesame salt, also called gomashio, on top of rice and vegetables to enhance the flavor. Gomashio is best made fresh every two weeks, using roasted black or tan sesame seeds, with a ratio of twenty parts sesame seeds to one part sea salt. Black sesame seeds, which contain a higher concentration of minerals compared to tan sesame seeds, support the kidney and help strengthen hair and bones.

Pickles

Pickles stimulate the production of hydrochloric acid and enzymes for improved digestion, help neutralize acidity, improve mental clarity, and provide a source of beneficial bacteria for the intestines. Pickles may be homemade or bought in the refrigerated section of the store. Avoid pasteurized pickles, which are cooked and no longer contain live beneficial bacteria. If pickles are too salty, rinse off salt or soak in cold water to remove surface salt. Use ½ tablespoon pickles at lunch and ½ tablespoon at dinner.

Beverages

Drink a comfortable amount daily (3–5 cups a day, including home remedies, but not soup) and whenever thirsty. Beverages that are for daily consumption are kukicha twig, roasted barley, and roasted brown rice tea. Avoid iced or icy cold drinks, but slightly chilled beverages are appropriate in warm weather.

Desserts

Fruit is a healthy choice for dessert, which is eaten in small amounts and in season, depending on your health condition. A little fresh or dried fruit cooked with a pinch of sea salt is best to balance natural sugars. If you live in temperate climates, reduce or limit raw fruit, which is very cooling. However, you can eat fresh seasonal northern climate fruit in summer, and use a pinch of salt to balance natural sugar. Since fruit juice is very concentrated, it should be used in moderation, depending on health, and use fresh fruit juice only, rather than frozen, pasteurized, or concentrated.

An alternative to fruit to satisfy sweet cravings is sweet vegetables. You can even make fresh carrot juice or a sweet vegetable drink, which is a tea, made by simmering sweet vegetables in water. A substitute for fruit jam is sweet vegetable jam, which is made by cooking sweet vegetables several hours over a low flame to make a thick paste that resembles vegetable purée.

Grain-based sweeteners are amasake, barley malt, and brown rice syrup. When substituting a liquid sweetener, such as brown rice syrup, for 1 cup granulated sugar, use 1¼ cup liquid sweetener and reduce liquid by ¼ cup (except oil). Apple juice, apple cider, and apple sauce can also be used as sweeteners for desserts. Good quality desserts taken 2–3 times a week in moderation include:

- Squash pudding
- Puréed chestnuts
- Amasake pudding
- Rice pudding (or sweet brown rice)
- Aduki kanten
- Fruit kanten

If your health condition permits, baked soft desserts such as apple pie and pear crisp and baked hard, dry desserts such as cookies, muffins, and cake are fine, but should be eaten in moderation.

Snacks

Healthy on-the-go snacks help reduce cravings between meals and keep your energy level elevated and your mind alert. Low in fat and high in nutrients, healthy snacks with whole grains contain complex carbohydrates instead of simple sugars like candy bars and soft drinks. Baked, hard, or puffed snacks are best avoided, but if craved, eaten in moderation once a week. Soft macrobiotic snacks for use daily include:

- Rice balls
- Noodles
- Corn on the cob
- Sushi
- Mochi
- Chickpea spread (hummus)
- Leftovers
- Vegetable aspic (kanten)

FACT

Obesity is a health problem for children and teenagers. According to data from National Health and Nutrition Examination surveys (1976–1980 and 2003–2006), the prevalence of obesity has increased from 5 percent to 12.4 percent for children aged 2–5 years, from 6.5 percent to 17 percent in those aged 6–11 years, and from 5 percent to 17.6 percent in those aged 12–19 years.

Incorporating snacks into your meal plan helps you prepare healthy small meals ahead of time, rather than waiting until hunger strikes. Studies on obesity show that eating frequent small meals lessens the strain on your liver, while controlling blood glucose levels and fat accumulation. Clearly, the health benefits of spreading energy intake over several small meals outweigh those of a few large ones.

Using Leftovers

Leftovers are the saving grace for staying within a macrobiotic meal plan with minimal effort. The extra food at dinner has new life as leftovers to use for breakfast and lunch the next day. If you are too busy to cook or you forgot to do your meal plan, you can still create easy and quick 10–15 minute meals (Table 4–7) to get you through the day. With luscious flavor and versatility, leftover grains, beans, and vegetables transform an ordinary meal into a new masterpiece.

Incorporating Cooking into Your Busy Life

The time-saving aspect of eating out can seem attractive on your busy schedule. However, cooking homemade macrobiotic meals has the advantages of being less expensive, better quality, and customizable. Making a meal from scratch requires planning and preparation, which is as important as the cooking itself in the overall process. To make the most of your time in the kitchen, remember the three "PREs" of preparation: presoak, prepare, and precook.

Presoak

Soak grains, beans, and dried vegetables (dried daikon, dried mushrooms, etc.) overnight so that they are ready to use when you prepare the meals. Reserve two to three bowls just for soaking, and keep them filled at all times. Schedule pickling of sauerkraut or other pickles at regular intervals to have an ongoing supply available for meals. Soaking items and pickles can be kept at room temperature away from sunlight, but refrigerate them to slow down fermentation until they are ready to use.

QUESTION

Is it necessary to soak grains before using them?
Soaking grains for at least 6–8 hours makes them more digestible and helps to dissolve phytic acid, an anti-nutrient found in grains, beans, nuts, and seeds. Phytic acid prevents the body from absorbing nutrients and can lead to mineral deficiency. Once phytic acid has been neutralized, the soaking water may be used to cook the grain.

Prepare

Consider the cooking time for each ingredient, and begin cooking foods that take the longest, such as beans and rice, first. Pressure cookers, which can conveniently shorten the cooking time for beans and rice, are often turned on first. In the meantime, prepare your vegetables by cutting them into various appealing shapes to balance the energy of the season. Vegetables cut into thin matchsticks work best for short-cooked sautés and salads in summer. However, in winter, cutting vegetables into large chunks is more appropriate for long-cooked soups and stews.

ALERT

In studies done in the former Soviet Union, serious health problems were associated with the consumption of microwaved food. The Soviets found that microwaving food significantly reduces the nutritional content of the food. Microwaved food was also found to promote emotional problems, cancer, heart disease, lymphatic disorders, digestive problems, blood and immune abnormalities, permanent brain damage, and hormonal imbalances.

Precook

Some recipes have multiple steps that involve precooking foods before mixing them with other ingredients. Set aside a block of time perhaps on the weekend to precook grains, beans, and dressings for quick meals during the week. Or make extra food at dinner and store precooked foods until you are ready to cook the remaining ingredients. Precooked rice and beans can be used as a base for salads, burgers, soups, burritos, loaves, and casseroles. Even precooked tempeh can be added to sandwiches, grains, beans, and vegetables. Blanched, roasted, steamed, and sautéed vegetables can also be added to fried rice, soups, salads, casseroles, noodles, nori rolls, and sauces. Caramelizing onions and mushrooms enhances their mouthwatering flavor before cooking them with other ingredients.

Children have wild imaginations and approach cooking as if they were playing a game. Likewise, you can bring imagination into the kitchen playground where you add this secret ingredient into each dish you create. As an intuitive cook, the best dishes are the ones that you create on the spur of the moment, using only a few ingredients at hand. Feel free to experiment with your foods, as you are limited only by your imagination. This is your recipe for success.

CHAPTER 5

Foods to Reduce or Avoid

Imagine putting your hands in the earth; planting seeds; watching plants mature; picking ripe fruits, vegetables, and herbs; and then creating delectable family meals. Developing an intimate connection with nature can help you understand the energy of food in a deeply personal way. As you develop your intuition, you may even find that some foods, such as sugar, meat, and dairy, have extreme energy and are best used in moderation. You may even wish to reduce or avoid these extreme foods to help make the transition process easier as you take the steps toward a macrobiotic lifestyle.

Nightshades

Nightshades are any of several plants belonging to the genus *solanum*. Some nightshade plants are eggplants, potatoes, red or green peppers, tobacco, and tomatoes. Nightshades, which are high in potassium, have an expansive, cooling effect on the body and can help balance the contracting, warming energy of meat. For example, yang, heavy, salty meat and yin, expansive potatoes are often eaten together. However, without meat to counterbalance the yin effects of nightshades, vegans can become weak and depleted from overconsumption of nightshades. If you are following a macrobiotic diet, locally grown nightshades, such as tomatoes, peppers, eggplant, and potato, are best eaten in moderation in the height of summer or in tropical climates.

The chemical and energetic qualities of nightshades produce extreme, expansive effects on the body. These effects include expanding and weakening bones, joints, teeth, gums, and organs, especially for those in weakened conditions. Besides being extremely yin, nightshades contain protein-like compounds called alkaloids (solanine in potatoes and eggplant, tomatine in tomatoes) which can cause calcium depletion and arthritis inflammation. Some nightshades, like tobacco, contain alkaloids (like nicotine) that are also stimulating and addictive.

FACT

According to statistics compiled by the National Center for Chronic Disease Prevention and Health Promotion, by 2005 an estimated 46 million adults in the United States reported a doctor-diagnosed form of arthritis, rheumatoid arthritis, gout, lupus, or fibromyalgia. By 2030, an estimated 67 million adult Americans are projected to be diagnosed with arthritis.

Potatoes

Potatoes in particular contain high levels of simple carbohydrates (starches), which make them taste good and raise blood sugar levels at the same time. People who are hypoglycemic can be attracted to potatoes to relieve symptoms of low blood sugar levels. Potatoes also help to counterbalance overly salted conditions. (Gourmet chefs know to add potatoes to soup that has been oversalted.) Because of their expanded, watery, yin nature, potatoes have a loosening effect on the large intestine and brain. This effect can contribute to mental dullness, scattered thinking, and inability to pay attention. Good substitutes for potatoes are sweet potatoes, sunchokes (Jerusalem artichokes), celery root, and rutabagas. (Refer to Chapter 3 Table 3-4 for possible vegetable substitutions.)

ALERT

Some herbal supplements or teas contain stimulants that are used to help boost the immune system. Examples of stimulating ingredients are tobacco, Deadly Nightshade (belladonna or mandrake), Echinacea, Kangaroo Apple, bittersweet, astragalus, ginseng, Jerusalem Cherry, and horse nettle. However, overstimulating an already weakened immune system with strong stimulants can be further depleting.

Tomatoes

Tomatoes are very cooling and have the ability to dissolve excess fatty deposits in the liver and other parts of the body. In fact, this extreme food is often used to counterbalance prostate cancer, which is a yang-type condition that can be caused by overconsumption of extreme yang fatty animal products. Because the alkaloid tomatine in tomatoes can cause calcium to be released from the bones, tomatoes are often craved by pregnant women to stimulate calcium release into the bloodstream for development of the fetus. However, if overdone, this calcium depletion can lead to osteoporosis in older adults. To substitute for tomatoes in a dish, you can make a sauce with beets, carrot, and red onion cooked together with a little umeboshi paste (Mock Tomato Sauce, page 187).

Dairy Products

Each species produces milk that is appropriate nutritionally and energetically for their growing offspring. Because cow's milk is not designed for human consumption, excess dairy products can create mucous stagnation that blocks energy from flowing through the body. Dairy products that are more yin and expanded (milk) tend to accumulate in the upper part of the body, such as the lungs and sinuses. In contrast, dairy products that are more yang and dense (cheese) tend to accumulate in the lower part of the body and reproductive organs. Overall, the excessive use of milk products can contribute to weakened immune system, constitution, and intuition.

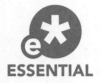

ESSENTIAL

Human milk is the perfect food for a growing baby. Besides containing essential vitamins and minerals in the appropriate amounts, breast milk has nonnutritive substances that are important in conferring immunity to the baby. Immune enhancers, antimicrobials, and inflammation soothers in breast milk give breastfed babies a health advantage over formula-fed babies.

Milk

Dairy products, cow's milk in particular, were considered to be the perfect food, as they contain a similar amount of lactose as human milk. Lactase is an enzyme that breaks down lactose in milk and dairy products. However, the majority of the world's population ceases to produce lactase after four years of age. If lactose builds up in the large intestine, it can ferment and react with many types of bacteria present. Bacteria in the large intestine then convert lactose into carbon dioxide and lactic acid, which can create mucus in the lung and produce acidic blood. This highly acidic blood is buffered by calcium released from bones, which can lead to osteoporosis.

ALERT

Although milk is high in calcium, calcium in milk may not be easily absorbed, and high amounts of acidic protein called casein may actually cause bone loss. Casein is a sticky, indigestible protein in milk that can form fatty cysts and tumors. Because calcium is bonded to casein as calcium caseinate, calcium itself can be difficult to absorb.

Good substitutions for milk are nut and grain milks, such as hazelnut milk, almond milk, oat milk, and rice milk. Puréeing soups or adding tahini or other nut butters can make a dish creamy instead of adding cream itself. Arrowroot or kuzu used to thicken sauces and gravies can also mimic the consistency of cream.

Butter

In traditional cultures, butter is considered to be a neutral fat, because it contains saturated fatty acids that are stable to heat, light, and oxygen. However, these saturated fatty acids can also make butter difficult to digest. Excess consumption of butter can also create mucus accumulation in the lungs and the heart. As a result, this area can become insulated from emotional experiences. In this way, butter and other dairy products can play a role in holding on to the past, resentments, and negative memories.

Olive oil and sesame oil are energetically balanced oils that are good substitutes for butter. Use these oils for cooking over low to medium flames, so as not to denature the oils. For baking or high-heat cooking, you can use sunflower, safflower, or grapeseed oil. Coconut butter and coconut oil, which come from tropical climates, are very yin compared to olive and sesame oil, but they can be used on occasion for baking in place of butter.

FACT

Stress causes cravings for sugar and high-fat food, both of which can enhance mood. In fact, casein in dairy products has a similar shape to beta-endorphins and stimulates the same pleasure receptors in the brain. A brain chemical called galanin also works together with endorphins for the pleasure response. Galanin triggers ice cream cravings, while endorphins make the experience pleasurable.

Cheese

The lactase in ripened cheese is converted into simple sugar by bacteria used in the cheese-making process. Cheese is compressed curds, containing concentrated casein and fat, which is much more acidic than milk. The yin, expanded nature of soft cheese softens and fattens the body, producing occlusions and coolness in the body. Hard cheese is very yang in comparison, because it is aged and dense. Whereas hard cheese contributes to kidney and gallstones, soft cheese contributes to pale skin and water retention.

You can recreate the consistency of cheese by stirring grated mochi into a hot dish, such as beans or sauce. Tofu Sour Cream (page 85) is an alternative to cream cheese, sour cream, or yogurt. It is made by blending tofu, rice or almond milk, lemon juice, sweet white miso, and umeboshi plum paste. (Look for Nigari Tofu and similar tofu products that are handmade in the traditional way using organic whole soybeans. Use tofu in moderation as garnish or in small portions, since overconsumption of tofu can weaken the intestines and kidneys.)

Ice Cream

Ice cream or frozen milk brings cooling yin energy into an overly heated body. However, often used as a comfort food, ice cream can create stagnation while covering up emotions, such as passion, compassion, and warmth. Frozen rice milk desserts (including Rice Dream products) are a good substitute for ice cream. Frozen juice bars or amasake are other healthy desserts that can replace ice cream.

Processed Soy Products

Soy products, including tofu, soymilk, and tempeh, are made from yellow soybeans, which have yin cooling energy. Tofu, in particular, can be used to calm stomach inflammation and neutralize toxins. Traditionally, tofu was used in Japan in small amounts cooked in miso soup, rather than as a main protein source. Today, large amounts of processed soy products are consumed in the Western diet, which can deplete chi and weaken the body. For instance, some soy products, such as imitation cheese, soy hot dogs, and soy frozen desserts, are highly processed and contain soy protein isolate or soy lecithin (used as emulsifiers), which are difficult to digest. These processed soy products can also create mucous stagnation in the kidneys and reproductive organs. The best way to consume yellow soybeans is in fermented form, which is less yin and more digestible. Fermented soy products include tempeh, miso, shoyu, tamari, and natto.

Tempeh is a fermented whole soybean product that is traditionally eaten in hot places. Because it is the least processed among soy products, it is more digestible and less yin than other soy products. The fermentation process for tempeh and miso also reduces levels of phytoestrogens and substances in soybeans that block thyroid function, mineral absorption, and glucose uptake in the brain. If homemade, tempeh can also be a valuable source of vitamin B12. Because of its heavy, dense, meaty quality, tempeh is a good substitute for meat in stews and sandwiches.

In Japan, black soybeans are considered the crown prince of all soybeans. Black soybeans are easier to digest than the yellow variety and considered to be medicinal for the spleen, kidney, and reproductive organs. They can even help cleanse an overly yang condition from too much animal food and fish. Black soybeans are especially beneficial for relieving contracted intestines and discharging baked flour products from the kidney. Black soybean tea can also help relieve problems associated with weak kidneys, such as spasms and cramps, inflammations, and chronic cough. As a good source of fat, calcium, and protein, they can further stimulate breastfeeding, regulate menstrual cycles, and reverse osteoporosis.

Tropical Foods

Foods grown in hot, tropical climates include tropical fruits and hot spices. Tropical foods have extreme yin energy compared to foods grown in a four-season climate. They are used to cool down bodies with excess heat, especially those of meat eaters.

Tropical Fruits

Tropical fruits, such as orange, papaya, mango, grapefruit, and banana, are more sensitive to growing conditions than most temperate climate fruits. (Temperate climate fruits, such as apple, pear, peach, plum, and berries, are those that are grown in a four-season climate.) Because tropical fruits have yin energy and cool down the body, they can put out the digestive fire (weaken digestion). People who are underactive or have weak digestion are unable to balance this cooling energy. A hot, tropical climate helps to balance a diet consisting of large quantities of fruit (sometimes in the form of smoothies, shakes, or juices). However, over the long term, if excessive fruit is absorbed into the bloodstream as sugar, and it is not burned off, fatigue and deficient chi can result.

ALERT

Tropical fruits, especially bananas, are also higher in sugar than temperate climate fruits. This high sugar content can contribute to acidic blood, mineral loss, and weakness in the kidney and reproductive organs. If the liver is overworked, high quantities of sugar from tropical fruits are also converted by the body into fat.

Locally grown fruit is easiest to assimilate and balance energetically. There are three ways to eat fruit: raw, dried, and cooked. Raw fruit is very cooling to the body and is also difficult to digest. Drying fruit concentrates the sugars, making this form difficult to balance energetically and biochemically. Cooking fruit with a pinch of salt helps to balance its yin cooling energy, makes it easier to digest, and is the best way to eat fruit.

Hot Spices

Hot spices, including hot chili pepper, have yin, upward, rising chi and help cool down the body in hot climates near the equator. Hot spices can also spark digestive fire (increase digestion), increase heart rate, and activate circulation. This is how hot spices induce perspiration, which helps to cool off the body. Meat eaters who have excessive heat can balance their yang energy with spicy foods. Vegetarians, however, are unable to balance the excess yin energy of hot spices, which can weaken their body and deplete their condition. As an alternative, herbs are milder for vegetarians to use in warm seasons. Sweet spices, such as cardamom and ginger, are also not as cooling to the body as hot spices.

Sugar

In prehistoric times, natural carbohydrates came from fruits, honey, bark, leaves, and grains in an unrefined form. Because natural sweets are seasonal, these foods were eaten in warm weather. Today, sugar or simple carbohydrates can come in many forms, including glucose, fructose, dextrose, sucrose, and lactose. Simple sugars elevate mood by raising neurotransmitter serotonin levels. Some foods that contain high amounts of simple sugars are alcohol, white flour products, white potatoes, and white rice. These products create sticky, mucous stagnation in the lung and large intestine, which can disrupt circulating chi and interfere with your intuition.

QUESTION

Can I substitute artificial sweeteners for sugar?
Artificial sweeteners, like saccharin and aspartame, are extreme yin chemicals that can disrupt nervous function and destroy brain cells. Artificial toxins are also cleansed by the liver, a process that uses your energy reserves and weakens your body overall. These toxic chemicals can also make you ungrounded and interfere with your intuition.

Refined Sugar

Refined sugar is a crystalline substance made from tropical sugar cane and sugar beet. The refining process strips sugar of its fiber, protein, vitamins, and minerals. This uses up the body's stores of vitamins, minerals, and enzymes to extract energy from the simple carbohydrates. Sugar has yin, cooling energy and balances yang meat diets. However, it can create imbalance in the body when eaten in excess or when the body is already in a weakened state. It suppresses the immune system, raises blood sugar levels, weakens digestion, and can cause acidic blood. In order to buffer this acidity, the body leeches calcium from bones, which can cause osteoporosis and kidney stones. Excessive consumption of sugar has also been linked to type-2 diabetes, obesity, and tooth decay.

Alcohol

Alcohol that is fermented from fruit, such as wine, is more yin than grain fermented beverages, like beer, sake, or whiskey. Meat eaters often seek to balance their overly yang condition with yin energy from alcohol. Alcohol goes directly into the bloodstream and, along with caffeine and nicotine, bypasses the blood-brain barrier (a network of blood vessels and cells that functions to filter blood passing into the brain). That is why these stimulants can affect the brain so quickly. Some effects of excess alcohol consumption are problems with walking, blurred vision, slurred speech, slowed reaction times, and memory loss. Alcoholics are often hypoglycemic and crave alcohol to relieve their low blood sugar levels. Kuzu tea counteracts the yin effects of alcohol (and alcoholism) by bringing downward, gathering energy to the intestines.

Energetically balanced whole grains contain complex carbohydrates that keep blood sugar levels steady. In the process of making sweeteners, these whole grains are turned into simple sugars. Although whole grain sweeteners are more yin than whole grains, these sweeteners are not as extremely yin as refined sugar. Good sugar substitutes, made from whole grains, include barley malt syrup, brown rice syrup, and amasake. Other healthy alternatives to sugar include:

- Granulated dried fruit (date sugar), maple sugar, and maple syrup are more yin compared to whole grain sweeteners, but they can be used in moderation in warm weather.
- In baked goods, puréed chestnuts or sweet potatoes are other good alternatives to sugar.
- Raisins or fruit-sweetened dried cranberries can add sweetness to desserts without adding sugar or another sweetener.
- Apple juice or apple sauce can also be used in baked recipes requiring sugar, if another liquid (except oil) is reduced to keep amounts proportional.

Refer to the Chapter 4 Supplement Dishes section for additional tips on desserts and liquid equivalent measurements for sugar substitutions. As you reduce the amount of sugar in your diet, your taste buds may become more sensitive to sweet taste, and you may prefer the natural balanced sweetness of whole grains.

Caffeine

Caffeine is a psychoactive drug found in more than sixty plants, where it acts as a natural pesticide. Coffee, tea, and soft drinks are popular beverages that can contain caffeine. Like nicotine, caffeine is an addictive plant alkaloid that is also a stimulant. Caffeine activates the adrenals to produce the "fight or flight" response. Increased stress hormones can also give you a feeling of euphoria, because they increase the need for neurotransmitter serotonin in the brain. However, like a roller coaster of extreme highs and lows, when caffeine wears off and serotonin levels decrease, a "crash" (irritability, anxiety, depression, and lack of concentration) can follow. Because it contains extreme yin, upward rising energy, overuse of caffeine can also deplete vital energy in vegans.

ESSENTIAL

Studies show that long-term coffee drinkers have a higher risk of health problems. Caffeine in coffee can cause increased heart rate, insomnia, and nervousness. Overconsumption of coffee has also been linked to mineral loss (osteoporosis), calcification of soft tissues, hardening of the arteries, arthritis, and kidney stones.

Kukicha twig tea is a Japanese green tea blend of twigs, stalks, and stems and has 90 percent less caffeine than traditional teas. Other alternatives to caffeinated teas are roasted barley tea and roasted brown rice tea. Grain coffee, which is made from roasted chicory, barley, beetroot, rye, and malted barley, is a good substitute for coffee. Herbal coffee, which is made from herbs, grains, fruits, and nuts, is also roasted, ground, and brewed to resemble coffee without the caffeine.

Meat

Traditional cultures worked outside and ate dense animal food that was burned off with a highly active lifestyle. They also ate wild grazing animals that were low in fat. Because most animals today eat grains and live in stalls, animal products, such as beef, pork, and lamb, are high in cholesterol and saturated fat. Most animals are also killed inhumanely and contain stress hormones, as well as pesticides, antibiotics, and growth hormones in their bloodstream.

Animals are warm and full of dense, contracted energy compared to the cool energy of plants. Yang animal foods gather energy and nutrients and stabilize the body and mind. This creates strength in the organs and body. However, overconsumption of extreme yang foods, such as meat, can create stagnation; a hard, tight, stiff body; and a craving for yin foods, such as sugar. Highly dense yang meat gives a jolt to the kidney and reproductive organs, increasing sex drive temporarily. However, eventually this extreme contracting energy, as well as the accumulation of saturated fat, can weaken these organs. Meat also produces strong acids in the body, which can also cause mineral depletion, as your body releases mineral stores to buffer this acidity.

ALERT

The process of curing meat with salt, nitrites, and smoking makes meat even more yang and contracted. Nitrites are preservatives, which give cured meats, such as beef jerky, hot dogs, bacon, sausage, and lox, their pink or red color. Because nitrites are also precursors to compounds called nitrosamines, which can promote cancer, look for nitrite-free cured meats.

Although it has cholesterol, fish is low in saturated fat compared to other animal products. To balance the yang contracting energy of fish, add plenty of greens, which have yin upward energy. Also, serve fish with lemon or pungent foods, such as raw grated daikon, ginger, or horseradish, to help dissolve oils. Good substitutes for meat are seitan, tempeh, and mushrooms, which can add a meaty, dense flavor to stews and gravies.

Processed Foods

Processed foods are transformed in some way from their natural state for many reasons, such as convenience and safety. Methods of processing include canning, freezing, refrigeration, dehydration, and aseptic processing (pasteurization). While some processed foods, like dehydrated fruit, are close to their natural state, other processed foods may contain artificial flavors, monosodium glutamate (MSG), trans fats, and preservatives. Some processed foods, like white flour products (white bread), are even fortified and enriched to add vitamins and minerals lost during the refining process.

White flour in particular lacks fiber and becomes sticky in the intestines. This weakens the large intestine and creates constipation as well as clogged thinking.

ALERT

While supplements can be beneficial to some people, it is far better to get vitamins and minerals from natural foods. In fact, the American Dietetic Association, the American Medical Association, and the National Institutes of Health all recommend calcium-rich foods rather than pills as calcium sources.

Processed and refined foods and supplements, although derived from whole foods, do not retain the same energy as whole foods that contain all the essential nutrients in balanced proportions to harmonize with the body's needs. Eating seasonal, locally grown food also allows the body to adapt to the climate and environment and become more energetically balanced. However, eating processed foods that are inappropriate for the climate and region often leads to weakness in the organs, so that the body becomes more susceptible to disease.

Because whole foods are unprocessed, they are a more natural way of eating. When you eat fresh, vibrant whole foods, you radiate life energy. This energy not only revitalizes you, it also helps you connect with nature in a deeper, more meaningful way.

CHAPTER 6

Appetizers and Snacks

Squash and Sweet Potato Dumplings

These dumplings are healing snacks for diabetes and hypoglycemia. Add gravy or ginger shoyu dipping sauce. Dumpling wrappers can be purchased at Asian markets.

INGREDIENTS | SERVES 2

1¾ pounds sweet potatoes, peeled
1¾ pounds butternut squash, peeled
1½ cups water
Sweet white miso, to taste
Lime juice, to taste
50 round dumpling wrappers
¼ cup safflower oil

Chewing

Proper chewing is as important to a meal as cooking. Chewing stimulates digestive enzymes, which alkalinize acidic foods, like brown rice. Put your chopsticks or fork down between bites. As you chew, take five in-breaths and five out-breaths. This ensures that you chew ideally between 50–100 times for each bite.

1. Chop sweet potatoes and squash into small cubes. Place sweet potatoes, squash, and water in a saucepan, and bring to a boil. Steam until vegetables are soft, about 15–20 minutes. Mash vegetables thoroughly with a masher or pass them through a food mill into a large bowl. Season to taste with sweet white miso and lime juice.

2. Place stack of wrappers on a plate and cover with a damp cloth to prevent them from drying out. Place a wrapper in the palm of one hand. Add 1 teaspoon of filling in center of wrapper. With a fingertip, dab one half of wrapper with a little water. Fold over other edge of wrapper and seal sides closed. Make 3 or 4 pleats along sealed edge. Place dumpling in a bowl and cover with a damp cloth. Repeat until filling is used up.

3. To cook dumplings, heat oil in a skillet. Pan fry dumplings until browned on each side, about 5 minutes.

PER SERVING   Calories: 94 | Fat: 2g | Sodium: 84mg | Carbohydrate: 17g | Fiber: 2g | Protein: 1g

Mushroom and Arugula Phyllo Triangles

Phyllo dough is thin sheets of unleavened flour dough used for making Greek pastries, like baklava, and appetizers. While traditional phyllo triangles use cheese as filling, this vegan version uses firm tofu.

INGREDIENTS | SERVES 24

8 ounces shiitake mushrooms, sliced

1 cup red onion, chopped

½ teaspoon dried tarragon

2 cloves garlic, minced

1 tablespoon plus ¾ cup safflower oil

12 ounces firm tofu

1 tablespoon sweet white miso

1 tablespoon lemon juice

⅛ teaspoon salt

3 bunches arugula, chopped

36 sheets phyllo dough, thawed in refrigerator

Tofu Sour Cream

Use this vegan sour cream as vegetable dip or to garnish bean burritos. Purée 12 ounces firm tofu with ¾ cup almond or rice milk, 1 teaspoon umeboshi paste, 1 tablespoon lemon juice, and sweet white miso, to taste.

1. In a skillet, sauté mushrooms, red onion, tarragon, and garlic in 1 tablespoon safflower oil. Sauté 10 minutes or until tender. Remove from heat.

2. Mix together tofu, miso, lemon juice, and salt. Add mushroom mixture to tofu mixture in bowl, and stir until combined.

3. Heat a large skillet over medium heat. Add 1 bunch arugula to pan; cook until wilted (about 7 minutes), stirring frequently. Drain. Repeat procedure with remaining arugula. Add arugula to mushroom tofu mixture in bowl. Stir until well combined.

4. Preheat oven to 400°F. Place 1 phyllo sheet on a large cutting board or work surface (cover the remaining dough to keep from drying). Lightly brush phyllo with safflower oil. Layer a sheet on top. Brush phyllo with more safflower oil. Layer one more sheet on top. Brush with more safflower oil. Cut stack lengthwise into four 3½"-wide strips.

5. Spoon about 1 rounded tablespoon arugula mixture onto one end of each strip. Fold one corner of the opposite end over mixture, forming a triangle. Keep folding back and forth into a triangle to the end of strip. Place triangles, seam-sides down, on a baking sheet. Lightly brush tops with safflower oil. Repeat procedure with remaining phyllo sheets and filling. Bake for 12 minutes or until golden.

PER SERVING Calories: 169 | Fat: 10g | Sodium: 168mg | Carbohydrate: 17g | Fiber: 1g | Protein: 4g

Roasted Wild Mushrooms, Walnut, and Lentil Pâté

Pâté can be eaten like hummus: as a dip for blanched vegetables, served on brown rice crackers, or spread on nori sushi. To make lentil loaf, omit oil, place lentil mixture into a greased loaf pan, and allow mixture to set as it cools. Slice and serve with gravy.

INGREDIENTS | SERVES 6

4 ounces fresh wild mushrooms, sliced

1 tablespoon sweet brown rice vinegar or balsamic vinegar

1 tablespoon safflower oil

1 tablespoon shallots, minced

Shoyu, to taste

1 tablespoon garlic, minced

1 cup French green or brown lentils

2 cups spring water

1 whole bay leaf

1 stamp-sized piece kombu

1 tablespoon tarragon

2 teaspoons barley miso

1 tablespoon umeboshi paste

3 tablespoons olive oil

½ cup walnuts, roasted and chopped

1. Preheat oven to 350°F. Mix mushrooms, sweet brown rice vinegar, safflower oil, shallots, shoyu, and garlic together on baking sheet. Roast in oven for 15 minutes.

2. In a small saucepan, add lentils and water. Bring to boil and skim off foam. Add bay leaf and kombu. Lower heat, and simmer, covered, for 45 minutes, adding more water as it evaporates. Remove bay leaf, drain lentils, and reserve cooking liquid.

3. In a suribachi or food processor, mix lentils, mushroom mixture, tarragon, miso, umeboshi paste, and olive oil, gradually adding cooking liquid to thin the pâté, if it becomes too thick. Stir in nuts.

PER SERVING Calories: 275 | Fat: 16g | Sodium: 265mg | Carbohydrate: 23g | Fiber: 11g | Protein: 11g

Red Lentil Pâté

Make easy red lentil pâté by cooking red lentils with sautéed onions and sweet vegetables. Add shoyu or sweet white miso at the end. Cook for 3 minutes. Add roasted and ground walnuts. Allow lentils to cool and spread on crackers or use in pita sandwiches. You can also coat them in corn meal and pan fry in oil.

Cucumber, Carrot, and Avocado Sushi Rolls

Sushi rolls are good for snacks or travel. Optional ingredients to include are nuts, seeds, tempeh, marinated shiitakes, umeboshi paste, mustard, noodles, pickled ginger and cucumber, or sauerkraut. Season brown rice with diluted umeboshi vinegar or sweet brown rice vinegar.

INGREDIENTS | SERVES 6

1 cup short grain brown rice

2 cups spring water

¼ teaspoon sea salt, divided

2½ tablespoons sweet brown rice vinegar

2 whole cucumbers, cut into matchsticks

1 large carrot, cut into matchsticks

6 sheets nori

2 whole avocados, sliced

1 tablespoon wasabi powder

Shoyu, to taste

Rice Balls

The rice ball is an energetically balanced food that is perfect for travel. A quarter of salted umeboshi plum is inserted into a ball of cooked brown rice, which is wrapped with antibacterial nori. Preserved in the center and protected on the periphery, a rice ball can be stored 3 days unrefrigerated.

1. Soak rice in water overnight in saucepan. Add ⅛ teaspoon salt. Bring to boil, lower heat, and simmer, covered, 45–50 minutes. Stir sweet brown rice vinegar into warm cooked rice. Allow rice to cool by spreading it out on sheet pan.

2. Sprinkle ⅛ teaspoon salt over cucumber to release water. Blanch carrots.

3. Place one sheet of nori shiny side down on the bamboo mat. Dampen hands with water. Pat a thin layer of rice onto nori, about ¼" thick, leaving ¼" plain nori border around the four edges. Place cucumber, carrot, and avocado together at the near edge.

4. Carefully and firmly roll up mat, dabbing the final edge of nori with a bit of water to seal. Place seam-side down. With a dampened bread knife, slice each roll into 6 segments. Clean off knife as you slice.

5. Serve with wasabi and shoyu. In a small saucepan, heat shoyu and a little water for 2–3 minutes. To prepare wasabi, mix 2 tablespoons wasabi powder with enough water to create a paste.

PER SERVING (WITHOUT SHOYU) Calories: 251 | Fat: 11g | Sodium: 73mg | Carbohydrate: 36g | Fiber: 8g | Protein: 6g

Veggie Greens Rolls

Veggie Greens Rolls are colorful with red and green leafy vegetables. Greens are good for discharging fat in the prostate and nourishing liver energy for women's health. A variation is to blanch kale instead of sauté. Adding a pinch of salt or umeboshi vinegar to cooking water conserves the color of cabbage.

INGREDIENTS | SERVES 4

1 medium carrot, cut into matchsticks

4 medium cabbage or collard leaves

2 cloves garlic, crushed

1 bunch red kale, chopped

1 teaspoon olive oil

¼ cup spring water

3 medium scallions, thinly sliced

4 tablespoons sauerkraut

Ume Plum Pumpkin Seed Sauce (page 180)

Variations of Greens Rolls

You can include various ingredients in Veggie Greens Rolls. Add grains, noodles, tempeh, marinated shiitakes, or nori. Add sauce inside the roll or on top, including pumpkin seed dressing, tahini, or kuzu sauce. Add sweetness to greens to lessen bitterness, such as parsnips or sweet white miso. Sour taste (mustard, umeboshi) also balances the sweetness of cabbage.

1. Blanch carrots 1 minute. Steam cabbage or collard leaves until tender and drain.

2. Sauté garlic and kale in oil until kale begins to wilt. Add water and cover. Cook until kale is tender, but retains a bright red color. Stir in scallions.

3. Place the cabbage leaves on a sushi mat. Layer kale on top of cabbage. Add 2 teaspoons of sauerkraut along the width of the roll. Place a few carrot sticks next to the sauerkraut.

4. Roll the vegetables using the sushi mat as a guide. Squeeze vegetables firmly in sushi mat to release excess water.

5. Slice the rolls into bite-sized pieces and serve with Ume Pumpkin Seed Sauce.

PER SERVING (WITHOUT SAUCE) Calories: 50 | Fat: 2g | Sodium: 93mg | Carbohydrate: 9g | Fiber: 2g | Protein: 2g

Humble Hummus

Traditional hummus recipes use tahini and chickpeas (garbanzos). For variety, add artichoke hearts, basil pesto, kalamata olives, sun-dried tomatoes, or roasted ground sesame seeds. Use heated herbed olive oil as garnish. Serve with blanched cut vegetables, crackers, or pita bread.

INGREDIENTS | SERVES 6

1 cup garbanzo beans, soaked

3 cups spring water

1 stamp-sized piece kombu

2 cloves garlic, crushed

3 medium scallions, finely chopped

2 tablespoons parsley, minced

2 teaspoons umeboshi paste

4 tablespoons lemon juice

1 tablespoon white miso

1 tablespoon olive oil

Cutting Techniques

To balance energy in a dish or gather energy for deeper healing, consider cutting techniques. To create balanced energy, cut vegetables toward center point: Cut greens starting from leafy tips toward stems. Cut roots starting from root end toward top. To strengthen intestinal energy, cut roots into matchsticks: Cut carrot or burdock on bias. Then thinly slice each section.

1. Drain beans. Place garbanzo beans and water in a pressure cooker. Bring to boil on a medium flame. Skim off foam. Add kombu. Cover, bring to pressure, lower heat, and pressure cook for 1 to 1¼ hours. Remove lid and allow beans to come to room temperature.

2. Strain out cooking liquid and set liquid aside. Purée garbanzo beans with a little cooking liquid. Add garlic, scallions, parsley, umeboshi paste, lemon juice, miso, and olive oil and purée, gradually adding a little cooking water to reach desired consistency. Add more umeboshi paste to taste if desired.

PER SERVING Calories: 156 | Fat: 4g | Sodium: 248mg | Carbohydrate: 23g | Fiber: 6g | Protein: 7g

Collard Dolmas Stuffed with Savory Brown Rice

Greek dolmas were traditionally made using grape leaves stuffed with seasoned white rice. Parsley, mint, pine nuts, yellow onion, spices, and orange zest are additional ingredients to include.

INGREDIENTS | SERVES 6

1 cup short grain brown rice

1¾ cups water or stock

Pinch salt

½ cup almonds, toasted

1 clove garlic, crushed

2 medium scallions, chopped

⅓ cup olive oil

Umeboshi vinegar, to taste

1 bunch collard greens

Lemon juice, to taste

Energy of Garlic

Garlic has a stimulating effect, which is appropriate in hot weather and to balance overconsumption of meat. However, garlic can be weakening for vegetarians, who need a more centered diet. Garlic pickled in miso for 10 days, which balances its extreme energy, is a better form for vegetarians to consume.

1. Soak rice overnight in water or stock in a pot. Add a pinch of salt. Bring to boil, lower heat, and simmer, covered, for 45–50 minutes. Remove from heat and set aside.

2. Finely chop almonds. Stir in almonds, garlic, scallions, and olive oil. Season with umeboshi vinegar, to taste.

3. Meanwhile, blanch collard greens for 1 minute. Drain and pat dry with a towel. Gently remove stems.

4. Lay out 1 collard leaf on plate. Place a scoopful of rice mixture in center of leaf. Fold sides in and roll up tightly. Repeat for remaining leaves.

5. To reheat, place in a steamer and steam for 5 minutes. Garnish with lemon juice.

PER SERVING Calories: 300 | Fat: 19g | Sodium: 26mg | Carbohydrate: 32g | Fiber: 5g | Protein: 6g

Vegan Tempeh "Meat" Balls

Vegan Tempeh "Meat" Balls are good as appetizers or made into burgers. Lentil purée and brown rice helps hold "meat" balls together. Tempeh balls can be baked or rolled in cornmeal and pan fried.

INGREDIENTS | SERVES 6

¼ cup onion, minced

1 clove garlic, crushed

¼ cup carrot, grated

¼ cup celery, minced

¼ teaspoon coriander

1 batch Marinated Tempeh (page 242)

½ cup cooked brown lentils

1½ cups cooked brown rice

¼ cup safflower oil

1. In a skillet, sauté onion, garlic, carrot, celery, and coriander until cooked. Crumble tempeh and add to the skillet with brown lentils and brown rice.

2. Form into balls. In a skillet, pan fry balls in oil until browned, about 10 minutes.

PER SERVING Calories: 280 | Fat: 18g | Sodium: 133mg | Carbohydrate: 21g | Fiber: 3g | Protein: 10g

Easy Marinade

Fish, portabella mushrooms, and tempeh can be marinated overnight or cooked in flavorful broth. Make an easy marinade by blending 1 part olive oil, 1 part shoyu, and 1 part sweet brown rice vinegar or balsamic vinegar. Include additional ingredients, like crushed garlic, lemon zest, sautéed onion, ginger, spices, or herbs.

Mushroom Cabbage Rolls

Cabbage rolls are warming snacks for late summer afternoons. Serve with Ume Plum Pumpkin Seed Sauce (page 180), Mock Tomato Sauce (page 187), or Shiitake Mushroom Onion Kuzu Gravy (page 184).

INGREDIENTS | SERVES 6

¾ cup brown rice, uncooked

1½ cups vegetable broth

2 pinches sea salt

¼ cup walnuts, toasted and chopped

1½ tablespoons safflower oil

¼ cup red onion, finely minced

2 cloves garlic, finely minced

1 cup fresh wild mushrooms, thinly sliced

2 tablespoons cilantro, finely chopped

1 pound green cabbage leaves, or Napa cabbage

Marinated Shiitakes

Marinated shiitakes are a delicious addition to sushi, pâté, vegetable rolls, or vegetable dishes. Soak fresh or dried shiitakes overnight in a mixture of one part shoyu, one part mirin, and one part water. Cook shiitakes in marinade until water is absorbed. Apple juice or brown rice syrup can be substituted for mirin.

1. Soak rice in broth overnight. In a medium saucepan, add rice, broth, and 1 pinch of salt. Bring to boil, lower heat, and simmer, covered, for 45 minutes.

2. Spread rice out in a wide bowl to cool slightly. While rice is cooking, dry roast walnuts in a skillet and chop them coarsely.

3. Heat 1 teaspoon oil in a medium skillet and sauté red onion, garlic, mushrooms, and 1 pinch of salt until mushrooms are soft. Stir mushroom-onion mixture, cilantro, and walnuts into cooled rice and set aside.

4. Steam the individual leaves of cabbage until soft and set aside to cool.

5. Heat 1 tablespoon oil in a skillet. Roll 2–3 tablespoons rice mixture into one cabbage leaf. Place each roll, seam-side down, in skillet. Pan fry cabbage rolls until crisp on bottom, about 5 minutes, and serve.

PER SERVING Calories: 122 | Fat: 7g | Sodium: 268mg | Carbohydrate: 13g | Fiber: 3g | Protein: 3g

Walnut and Chestnut Pâté

Walnuts are high in omega-3 fatty acids, which keep blood vessels flexible and support heart health. Chestnuts and walnuts are good for autumn cooking. Serve this pâté on brown rice crackers, toast, pita bread, steamed cabbage leaf, nori, or use as dip for blanched vegetables.

INGREDIENTS | SERVES 6

1 cup walnuts

Spring water, as needed

¼ cup carrots, finely grated

¼ teaspoon ginger juice

¼ cup fresh roasted chestnuts or Chestnut Purée (below)

Shoyu, to taste

1. Toast walnuts in skillet until lightly browned, about 8 minutes, and soak overnight in water to cover.

2. Drain walnuts. Mix remaining ingredients except shoyu with walnuts and purée. Season with shoyu, to taste.

PER SERVING Calories: 145 | Fat: 13g | Sodium: 7mg | Carbohydrate: 6g | Fiber: 1g | Protein: 3g

Chestnut Purée

Naturally sweet chestnuts can be made into purée for desserts and pâté. To make chestnut purée, soak 1 part dried chestnuts in 2 parts water overnight. Pressure cook or simmer 30–45 minutes until soft. Remove chestnuts and purée. Add tahini, nut butters, puréed soaked nuts (cashews, walnut), or barley malt.

CHAPTER 7

Good Morning Breakfasts

Brown Rice Porridge with Shiitakes and Miso

Brown Rice Porridge (ojiya in Japanese, juk in Chinese) is a healing congee that improves digestive function. You can simmer porridge over a low flame overnight instead of pressure cooking. If you include ojiya for breakfast, miso soup is not necessary.

INGREDIENTS | SERVES 2

½ cup yellow onion, diced

1 teaspoon sesame oil

2 dried shiitake mushrooms, soaked

2 cups water, including mushroom soaking water

1 cup cooked brown rice

1 stamp-sized piece kombu

½ cup celery, diced

Barley miso, to taste

¼ cup cilantro, chopped

1. In a skillet, sauté onion in sesame oil until translucent.

2. Remove stems from shiitakes and dice caps. In a pressure cooker, add water, brown rice, kombu, shiitake caps, celery, and onion. Cover, bring to pressure, lower heat, and cook 50 minutes.

3. Open cover, and remove a little porridge. Purée miso with porridge in suribachi bowl.

4. Season rest of porridge with barley miso purée. Simmer 3 more minutes.

5. Garnish with chopped cilantro.

PER SERVING Calories: 165 | Fat: 3g | Sodium: 119mg | Carbohydrate: 31g | Fiber: 4g | Protein: 3g

Washing Brown Rice

Washing brown rice can help you connect with nature. Pour cool water over grains in a bowl. Run your hands through them, and feel their texture. Observe their color variations. Raise a handful of grains to your nose and smell the aroma. Stir grains again and drain. Rinse grains until water drains clear.

Amazing Amaranth Porridge with Amasake

Like millet and quinoa, amaranth is a gluten-free, protein-rich, alkaline grain. When cooked, amaranth becomes creamy porridge, which nourishes heart health. Salty sour umeboshi plum also helps balance acidic blood. A little brown rice syrup, raisins, or amasake adds a touch of sweetness.

INGREDIENTS | SERVES 2

½ cup amaranth

1½ cups water

Pinch sea salt

Amasake, to taste

½ medium umeboshi plum

1. Pour amaranth and water in saucepan and soak overnight. Add pinch of salt. Bring to boil, lower heat, and simmer, covered, 30 minutes.

2. Let sit off heat 5 minutes. Add amasake to taste.

3. Garnish with umeboshi plum.

PER SERVING Calories: 180 | Fat: 3g | Sodium: 138mg | Carbohydrate: 32g | Fiber: 3g | Protein: 7g

Amazing Amasake Pancakes

Grains sweetened with amasake make delicious pancakes. To make Amazing Amasake Pancakes, mash 1 cup cooked grain (brown rice, millet, quinoa, couscous) with amasake, to taste. Add flour or arrowroot, as needed, to absorb moisture. Form mixture into four patties. Fry patties in 1 tablespoon safflower oil until browned on each side, about 10 minutes. Serve with Berry Lemon Sauce (page 100).

Soft Polenta and Peas

Fire energy of polenta helps discharge stagnation from overconsumption of eggs, which have a hardening effect on the pancreas and ovaries. You can also add sweet winter squash, carrots, corn, or lemon juice for variety.

INGREDIENTS | SERVES 2

1 cup corn grits
4 cups water
¼ teaspoon salt
½ cup fresh peas
Umeboshi plum paste, to taste
Gomashio, to taste

1. In a saucepan, toast corn grits until fragrant. Add water and salt. Bring to boil, lower heat, and simmer, covered, for 20 minutes. Stir polenta occasionally.

2. Add fresh peas and continue to cook 10 more minutes.

3. Season with umeboshi paste and gomashio, to taste.

PER SERVING Calories: 315 | Fat: 1g | Sodium: 337mg | Carbohydrate: 67g | Fiber: 3g | Protein: 9g

Millet Porridge with Vegetables

Creamy millet porridge cooked with sweet vegetables relaxes a contracted pancreas (and relieves hypoglycemia) caused by overconsumption of extreme yang foods (eggs, cheese, chicken, baked flour products). Mushrooms, marinated tempeh, or burdock can be added for a heartier stew.

INGREDIENTS | SERVES 6

2 cups millet, rinsed

6 cups water

¼ cup onion, diced

2 cloves garlic, crushed

1 teaspoon sesame oil

½ cup butternut squash, peeled

½ cup cabbage, chopped

¼ cup carrot, diced

1 teaspoon dried thyme

⅛ teaspoon salt

¼ cup parsley, chopped

1. In a Dutch oven, dry roast millet until fragrant and toasted. Add water and soak overnight.

2. In a skillet, sauté onion and garlic in oil until translucent.

3. Chop squash into small chunks. Add squash to millet along with sautéed onion and garlic and remaining ingredients, except parsley. Bring to boil, lower heat, and simmer, covered, 35 minutes.

4. Garnish with parsley.

PER SERVING Calories: 273 | Fat: 4g | Sodium: 64mg | Carbohydrate: 52g | Fiber: 7g | Protein: 8g

Energy of Millet

Millet is a round, hard, dense yellow grain eaten in cool climates. In contrast to brown rice, millet has no split in the center; millet is more contained, more round, and more whole. Because it is more yang than brown rice, millet absorbs more water. For 1 cup brown rice, use 1½–2 cups water, and for 1 cup millet, use 3 cups water.

Mochi Waffles with Berry Lemon Sauce

Because mochi is made by pounding sweet brown rice until grains are crushed, it contains downward contracting energy that strengthens intestinal function. The Berry Lemon Sauce is a healthy substitute for traditional syrups. You can also use jam, nuts, fruit, seeds, cinnamon, or amasake as toppings.

INGREDIENTS | SERVES 2

1 pound mochi
Berry Lemon Sauce, to taste (see below)
¼ cup pine nuts, toasted
1 small mint leaf
1 teaspoon orange zest

Berry Lemon Sauce

Delectable Berry Lemon Sauce makes a great topping for pancakes, mochi waffles, puddings, frozen rice milk desserts, and toast. Heat ½ cup brown rice syrup, 2 tablespoons water, 2 teaspoons lemon juice, and a pinch of salt. Turn off heat. Add ½ cup chopped fresh berries (strawberries, blueberries, raspberries).

1. Slice mochi into ¼" thick strips.

2. Place strips in hot waffle iron.

3. Cook until puffy and crispy.

4. Top with Berry Lemon Sauce.

5. Garnish with pine nuts, mint leaf, and orange zest.

PER SERVING, WITHOUT SAUCE   Calories: 613 | Fat: 16g | Sodium: 0mg | Carbohydrate: 116g | Fiber: 5g | Protein: 11g

Country Tempeh Sausages

Cholesterol-free vegan tempeh sausages go well with Buckwheat Pancakes (page 102). Tempeh sausages are a great addition to arame or hijiki dishes. Serve with gravy or ginger sauce, or use for sandwiches. Rice syrup or mirin can be substituted for apple juice.

INGREDIENTS | SERVES 4

8 ounces tempeh

½ cup spring water

1 tablespoon shoyu or tamari

¼ cup apple juice

1 tablespoon sesame oil

2 tablespoons sauerkraut

1 sheet nori, cut into fourths

¼ cup scallions, finely sliced

Cooking Tempeh

Cooking tempeh 20 minutes (steamed or simmered in water) helps remove its bitter flavor. You can also create a broth, gravy, or marinade to add flavor. Marinated tempeh can then be used in vegetable dishes or on its own seasoned with shoyu. Sautéing seasoned tempeh in oil balances its yin quality.

1. Slice tempeh into 1"-wide strips. Place tempeh, water, shoyu, and apple juice in a saucepan. Bring to boil, lower heat, and simmer, covered, 20 minutes.

2. Heat oil in a skillet. Pan fry tempeh on all sides, until browned.

3. Roll tempeh and sauerkraut in nori squares and garnish with scallions.

PER SERVING Calories: 152 | Fat: 10g | Sodium: 266mg | Carbohydrate: 8g | Fiber: 1g | Protein: 11g

Buckwheat Pancakes

Eaten in Russia and Poland, energizing and nutritious buckwheat is used in traditional dishes to provide warming energy for cold winter months. Buckwheat is high in magnesium and antioxidants, which can improve cardiovascular health and protect against heart disease.

INGREDIENTS | SERVES 4

1 cup buckwheat flour

½ cup spelt flour

1 teaspoon ground cinnamon

⅛ teaspoon salt

3 tablespoons safflower oil

1½ cups vegan milk

Berry Lemon Sauce (page 100), for garnish

Energy of Yeast and Leavening Agents

In commercial bread making, yeast was isolated from sourdough starter to increase bread size. Unlike natural sourdough starter, yeast has expansive yin effects that weaken the intestines, causing gas or constipation. Baking soda and baking powder also have yin effects and are not recommended on a healing diet.

1. In a large bowl, mix dry ingredients together. Mix wet ingredients together in a separate bowl. Pour wet ingredients into dry ingredients and mix. Cover bowl with moist towel, and let batter sit overnight at room temperature.

2. Brush bottom of skillet with safflower oil and heat over medium heat. Spread batter onto skillet, making a 4"-wide pancake. As bottom of pancake becomes browned, flip pancake over. When second side is browned, remove to a plate. Continue with remaining batter.

3. Serve with Berry Lemon Sauce.

PER SERVING, WITHOUT SAUCE Calories: 294 | Fat: 12g | Sodium: 80mg | Carbohydrate: 43g | Fiber: 6g | Protein: 6g

Soft Rice with Barley

Light, upward energy of spring barley helps dissolve animal protein and fat accumulations in the body from oily winter cooking. Barley water (yin, cooling) also helps dissolve nicotine (yang, contracting) from longtime smoking.

INGREDIENTS | SERVES 4

1 cup brown rice, rinsed
¼ cup barley, rinsed
6 cups spring water
⅛ teaspoon salt
½ cup walnuts, toasted
Umeboshi vinegar, to taste
¼ cup scallions, chopped
1 sheet nori, cut into strips

1. In a pressure cooker, add brown rice, barley, and water. Soak overnight.

2. Add salt. Cover, bring to pressure, lower heat, and pressure cook 50 minutes.

3. Chop walnuts. Add walnuts to grains. Season with umeboshi vinegar. Garnish with scallions and nori.

PER SERVING Calories: 311 | Fat: 11g | Sodium: 86mg | Carbohydrate: 47g | Fiber: 5g | Protein: 8g

Barley

The oldest known cultivated grain, barley comes in three forms: hulled, pearled, and hato mugi. Most natural hulled barley has the outer husk removed, keeping vitamin-rich endosperm and germ layers intact. Less nutritious pearled barley is polished, removing both endosperm and germ layers. Hato mugi (Job's tears) is wild grass with properties similar to barley.

Quinoa with Corn

Quinoa and corn both evoke feelings of peace and joy in the heart. Wholesome sweetness of corn is balanced with salty sour taste of umeboshi vinegar. Sweet squash and onion can also be included in this dish.

INGREDIENTS | SERVES 2

½ cup quinoa, rinsed

1 cup water

½ cup corn

Pinch sea salt

Toasted sesame oil, to taste

Umeboshi vinegar, to taste

1. In a saucepan, add quinoa, water, corn, and sea salt. Bring to boil, lower heat, and simmer, covered, 20 minutes.

2. Season with toasted sesame oil and umeboshi vinegar.

PER SERVING Calories: 190 | Fat: 3g | Sodium: 59mg | Carbohydrate: 35g | Fiber: 4g | Protein: 7g

Energy of Corn

Corn comes in two forms: fresh corn (vegetable) and maize (grain). Native Americans cooked maize as their staple grain in warm climates. Yang maize, rather than yin fresh corn, is best for strengthening the heart. Starchy fresh corn has more allergenic properties than maize and can affect diabetes and hypoglycemia.

Whole Oat Groats

High fat, warming whole oat groats are included in a building diet for growth or weight gain. Garnish with gomashio or shiso powder for healing instead of amasake, raisins, or jam. Rolled or steel cut oats, which are cracked and more yin than whole oats, are good for hot weather.

INGREDIENTS | SERVES 2

5 cups spring water
1 cup whole oat groats, rinsed
⅛ teaspoon sea salt
Gomashio, to taste
½ medium umeboshi plum

1. Add water to oats in a pressure cooker. Soak overnight.

2. Add salt. Cover, bring to pressure, lower heat, and pressure cook 50 minutes.

3. Add gomashio, to taste. Garnish with umeboshi plum.

PER SERVING Calories: 221 | Fat: 5g | Sodium: 242mg | Carbohydrate: 54g | Fiber: 8g | Protein: 14g

Great Grains

Millet Croquettes

Downward settling energy of millet supports digestive health. Leftover millet can be pan fried as is or breaded with corn meal or bread crumbs. Thicken watery millet with arrowroot or flour. Celery and arame can also be included. Serve with grated raw daikon.

INGREDIENTS | SERVES 6

1 cup millet

3 cups spring water

½ cup pumpkin seeds, toasted

½ bunch scallions, minced

½ bunch parsley, minced

1 small carrot, finely grated

Shoyu, to taste

¼ cup safflower oil

Cilantro Cashew Curry Sauce (below), for garnish

Cilantro Cashew Curry Sauce

This tasty sauce spices up grain burgers or blanched vegetables. Blend ¼ cup cashew butter, 1 tablespoon curry paste, 1½ tablespoons shoyu, and ¼ cup chopped cilantro with ¼–¾ cup water. To make curry paste, heat 2 teaspoons curry with 1 teaspoon olive oil. Experiment with various nut and seed butters and fresh herbs.

1. In a saucepan, dry roast millet over medium heat, stirring constantly, until fragrant, about 6 minutes. Remove from heat. Add water and soak millet overnight.

2. Bring to boil, lower heat, and simmer, covered, 30 minutes. Transfer to bowl.

3. Grind pumpkin seeds in suribachi or food processor. Add seeds, scallions, parsley, and carrot to millet. Mix ingredients and season with shoyu.

4. Form millet into croquettes. Heat oil in skillet and pan fry croquettes until browned on each side.

5. Serve with Cilantro Cashew Curry Sauce.

PER SERVING, WITHOUT SAUCE Calories: 313 | Fat: 19g | Sodium: 2mg | Carbohydrate: 29g | Fiber: 4g | Protein: 10g

Quinoa and Pumpkin Seed Pilaf

Heart healthy and nutritious quinoa is a gluten-free, alkaline grain. Any seasonal blanched vegetables can be used, including corn, broccoli, beets, green beans, and peas. You can also add sautéed mushrooms or marinated tempeh.

INGREDIENTS | SERVES 4

1 teaspoon olive oil
½ cup onion, diced
½ cup carrot, diced
¼ cup celery, diced
1 cup quinoa, rinsed
2 cups water or vegetable broth
⅛ teaspoon salt
¼ cup fresh parsley, finely chopped
1 teaspoon umeboshi paste
¼ cup pumpkin seeds, toasted
1 teaspoon tahini
½ teaspoon shoyu
Lemon juice, to taste

1. In a skillet, heat oil and sauté onion, carrot, and celery until onion is translucent.

2. In a saucepan, dry roast quinoa over low flame for 5 minutes until fragrant.

3. Add water or broth, onion, carrot, celery, and salt. Bring to boil, lower heat, and simmer, covered, 20 minutes.

4. Mix in remaining ingredients except lemon juice.

5. Add lemon juice, to taste.

PER SERVING Calories: 266 | Fat: 10g | Sodium: 222mg | Carbohydrate: 33g | Fiber: 5g | Protein: 11g

Brown Rice Burgers

This is a delicious way to prepare leftover grain. Make these ahead of time and store in refrigerator ready to heat. Toppings can include chopped toasted nuts, gomashio, sauerkraut, and shiso condiment. Serve with Shiitake Mushroom Onion Kuzu Gravy (page 184).

INGREDIENTS | SERVES 12

2 cups brown rice, rinsed

4 cups spring water

¼ teaspoon salt

1 tablespoon tahini

3 medium scallions, finely sliced

2 tablespoons umeboshi paste

¼ cup safflower oil

3 tablespoon tamari, optional

3 sheets nori, each cut into fourths, optional

Brown Rice

Brown rice comes in short-grain, medium-grain, and long-grain varieties. Cooked short-grain brown rice is sweet and glutinous, medium-grain is soft and moist, and long-grain is light and fluffy. Long-grain is best suited for hotter climates, medium-grain for warmer climates, and short-grain for temperate climates.

1. In a pressure cooker, soak rice overnight in water. Add salt and cover. Bring to pressure, lower heat, and pressure cook 50 minutes.

2. Let rice cool and stir in tahini and scallions. Wet hands and shape into balls. Dig a hole inside each one and insert ¼ teaspoon umeboshi paste. Flatten and shape into burgers.

3. Heat oil in skillet and pan fry each burger until browned on each side.

4. Optional: Season with tamari and wrap each burger with nori.

PER SERVING Calories: 166 | Fat: 6g | Sodium: 223mg | Carbohydrate: 25g | Fiber: 1g | Protein: 3g

Brown Rice with Dried Shiitakes

This recipe is perfect for cool fall weather. Downward gathering energy of brown rice improves intestinal function and helps ground you. Compared to boiled brown rice, pressure cooked brown rice is easier to digest, sweeter, more glutinous, more nutritious, and firmer.

INGREDIENTS | SERVES 6

2 cups brown rice, rinsed

3 dried shiitake mushrooms

3¾ cups water

¼ teaspoon salt

Gomashio, as needed

Seasoning Brown Rice

Brown rice can be seasoned in three ways: sea salt (⅛ teaspoon per cup brown rice), kombu (1 stamp-sized piece per cup brown rice), or umeboshi plum (½ plum per cup brown rice). All of these seasonings provide minerals, although kombu (yin) has the least amount of minerals and sea salt (yang) has the most.

1. In a pressure cooker, soak rice and mushrooms overnight in water. Add salt and cover. Bring to pressure, lower heat, and pressure cook 50 minutes.

2. Take out shiitakes and remove stem. Slice caps into thin strips. Add caps back to rice and stir. Serve with gomashio: ⅛ teaspoon per person.

PER SERVING Calories: 78 | Fat: 1g | Sodium: 101mg | Carbohydrate: 17g | Fiber: 1g | Protein: 2g

Brown Rice with Kidney Beans

Kidney beans are rich in folate and magnesium to support heart health. This satisfying dish includes traditional staples beans and grain cooked in a ceramic pot. When beans and grains are cooked together, beans adjust their cooking time to match that of grain.

INGREDIENTS | SERVES 4

¼ cup kidney beans

2½ cups spring water, plus enough to cover beans

1 cup brown rice, rinsed

1 stamp-sized piece kombu

Shoyu, to taste

Ohsawa Pot

An Ohsawa pot is a covered ceramic or glass pot (use a plate to cover) that fits inside a pressure cooker. Because the pot sits in water away from the flame, brown rice becomes fluffy, sweet, chewy, and easy to digest. This brown rice will be missing the metallic taste that comes from stainless steel. An Ohsawa pot can be used all year long.

1. In a bowl, soak kidney beans in water to cover overnight. In Ohsawa pot, soak brown rice in 2½ cups water overnight.

2. Discard bean-soaking water. Pour beans into saucepan and cover with fresh water. Bring to boil and skim off foam. Drain.

3. Add beans and kombu to rice and water in Ohsawa pot and cover. Fill a pressure cooker with 1½" water. Place a rack or two short chopsticks on the bottom. Place Ohsawa pot on rack or chopsticks.

4. Cover pressure cooker, bring to pressure, lower heat, and pressure cook 50 minutes.

5. Season with shoyu, to taste.

PER SERVING Calories: 187 | Fat: 1g | Sodium: 75mg | Carbohydrate: 39g | Fiber: 3g | Protein: 4g

Mushroom Polenta Burgers

Heart healthy Mushroom Polenta Burgers are delicious veggie burgers that can be made ahead of time and reheated. You can also include cooked wild rice, carrots, celery, spices, and herbs. Serve with Shiitake Mushroom Onion Kuzu Gravy (page 184).

INGREDIENTS | SERVES 4

1 teaspoon olive oil
½ cup onion, minced
1 clove garlic, crushed
½ cup fresh shiitakes, minced
1 teaspoon fresh sage, chopped
1 teaspoon fresh rosemary, chopped
5 cups water
2 cups cornmeal
¼ teaspoon salt
¼ cup safflower oil

1. In a skillet, heat olive oil and sauté onion and garlic until translucent. Add mushrooms, sage, and rosemary, and sauté until mushrooms are cooked through.

2. In a saucepan, bring water to boil. Add cornmeal, mushroom and onion mixture, and salt. Lower heat and continue stirring until water is absorbed.

3. Pour polenta into baking pan. Let cool in refrigerator.

4. Cut out circles, using cookie cutter or large glass jar.

5. Heat safflower oil in skillet and pan fry burgers until browned on both sides.

PER SERVING Calories: 444 | Fat: 16g | Sodium: 164mg | Carbohydrate: 67g | Fiber: 4g | Protein: 7g

Forbidden Rice with Edamame and Orange Zest

Once reserved for the emperor of China, forbidden rice was considered to be the finest quality rice. Nutty, chewy, dark purple grains are iron rich and considered a blood toner. Sautéed carrot matchsticks and broccoli florets can make great additions to this recipe.

INGREDIENTS | SERVES 4

½ cup forbidden rice, rinsed

1 cup spring water

1 teaspoon sesame oil

½ cup onion, diced

½ cup button mushrooms, diced

1/16 teaspoon salt

½ cup edamame, shelled

1 batch Orange Sesame Dressing (page 193)

1 teaspoon orange zest

Storing Brown Rice

Serve brown rice with a wooden paddle to scoop grain into a wooden or bamboo bowl. Stir grain to mix energies. Store grain, covered with a bamboo mat, in the pantry or on a kitchen counter for 2–3 days. Because vegetables decompose faster than grain, a dish of brown rice and vegetables needs to be eaten within 24 hours.

1. Soak rice overnight in water. In a skillet, heat oil and sauté onion until translucent. Add mushrooms and sauté until cooked through.

2. Add mushroom onion mixture and salt to rice and water in saucepan. Bring to boil, lower heat, and simmer, covered, 30 minutes.

3. Blanch edamame until tender. Mix edamame into rice.

4. Toss with Orange Sesame Dressing. Garnish with zest.

PER SERVING   Calories: 193 | Fat: 9g | Sodium: 334mg | Carbohydrate: 25g | Fiber: 4g | Protein: 6g

Vegetable Shepherd's Pie with Millet Crust

This vegan shepherd's pie layers textures, colors, smells, and flavors that combine into a delectable feast for the senses. Polenta or tortillas can be substituted for millet crust. Leftover vegetables can also be included.

INGREDIENTS | SERVES 4

1 cup millet, rinsed

7 cups spring water

2 cups sweet potatoes, peeled

2 cups cauliflower florets, blanched

2 cups green beans, blanched

1 batch Garbanzo Beans in Mushroom Gravy (page 149); Leek Almond Kuzu Gravy (page 185); Leek Tahini Ume Gravy (page 183); Tempeh with Arame, Shiitake, Onion Gravy (page 159); or Mock Tomato Sauce (page 187)

1 cup mochi, grated, optional

Millet

Grown in China, India, and Africa, millet is rich in complex carbohydrates and helps even out blood sugar levels. This makes it a good grain for diabetes and hypoglycemia. Millet also has an alkaline effect, which is good for acidic conditions like candida. Because it has gathering energy, there is no need to add salt when cooking millet.

1. Dry roast millet in saucepan until fragrant. Add 3 cups spring water and soak overnight. Bring millet and water to boil, lower heat, and simmer, covered, for 30 minutes.

2. Chop sweet potatoes into chunks. Bring 4 cups spring water to boil, add sweet potatoes, and boil until tender. Mash sweet potatoes.

3. Preheat oven to 350°F. Layer millet on bottom of baking pan. Layer cauliflower on top of millet. Layer green beans on top of cauliflower. Pour gravy or sauce on top of vegetables until gravy reaches halfway up vegetables. Layer sweet potatoes on top.

4. Bake until gravy or sauce bubbles, about 30 minutes.

5. Optional: Add grated mochi to vegetable layer. Prepare as usual.

PER SERVING (WITH GARBANZO BEAN IN MUSHROOM GRAVY RECIPE) Calories: 486 | Fat: 6g | Sodium: 691mg | Carbohydrate 93g | Fiber: 19g | Protein: 21g

Millet and Quinoa Pilaf with Burdock

Burdock's downward gathering energy strengthens the kidney and large intestine and adds meaty flavor to fluffy millet and quinoa. Matchstick carrots, corn, or green beans can also be included. Adding beets creates red pilaf that is colorful on the plate.

INGREDIENTS | SERVES 8

¾ cup millet, rinsed

3¾ cups spring water

½ cup burdock, cut into matchsticks

2 teaspoons sesame oil

½ cup onion, diced

½ cup carrot, cut into matchsticks

½ cup red quinoa, rinsed

⅛ teaspoon salt

¼ cup toasted walnuts, chopped

¼ cup parsley, minced

Energy of Roasting Millet

Millet can be dry roasted before cooking. Because millet is a yang grain, roasting contracts it even more. This is good for an overly expanded heart, which regulates contractions. Roasted millet absorbs more water during cooking. So, not only does roasting add bitter flavor, millet also becomes fluffier and softer.

1. Dry roast millet in saucepan until fragrant. Add water and soak overnight.

2. In a saucepan, sauté burdock in oil until soft, about 5 minutes. Add onion and carrot and sauté until onion is translucent.

3. Bring millet and water to boil, lower heat, and simmer, covered, 10 minutes.

4. Add quinoa, vegetables, and salt. Bring to boil, lower heat, and simmer, covered, 20 more minutes.

5. Mix walnuts into dish. Garnish with parsley.

PER SERVING Calories: 157 | Fat: 5g | Sodium: 47mg | Carbohydrate: 24g | Fiber: 3g | Protein: 4g

Mediterranean Brown Rice Salad

Warm Tuscan olive groves can be tasted in this salad, reminiscent of the Mediterranean. Brown rice salad is best served cold on a summer day. Additional ingredients to include are red onion, scallions, sun-dried tomatoes, parsley, sunflower seeds, and capers.

INGREDIENTS | SERVES 4

2 cups brown rice, cooked

½ cup black pitted olives, chopped

¼ cup carrots, grated

1 batch Basil Lemon Mustard Vinaigrette (page 199)

6 large lettuce leaves, romaine

¼ cup pine nuts, toasted

1. Mix brown rice, olives, and carrots together.

2. Add vinaigrette and mix. Roll in lettuce leaves with pine nuts.

PER SERVING Calories: 521 | Fat: 44g | Sodium: 210mg | Carbohydrate: 30g | Fiber: 4g | Protein: 5g

Three Grain Salad

Delicious Three Grain Salad makes a great addition to your lunch box. Just mix any three grains with your favorite dressing or vinaigrette: millet, brown rice, barley, quinoa, wheat berries, wild rice, bulgur, and couscous. Vegetables to add color and texture include green beans, carrot, scallion, red onion, parsley, and corn. Include nuts and seeds for crunch.

CHAPTER 9

Voluptuous Vegetables

Glazed Baby Carrots

Early harvest Nantes carrots are true baby carrots bred to be picked when tender. Rich in beta-carotene, they come in rainbow colors—yellow, white, purple, orange, and scarlet. Downward gathering energy of baby carrots nourishes intestinal function and grounds the lower region of the body.

INGREDIENTS | SERVES 6

1 bunch rainbow baby carrots (about 3 cups)

1 teaspoon olive oil

½ cup water

2 teaspoons brown rice syrup, or to taste

½ teaspoon tamari, or to taste

Juice of ½ lime

1 tablespoon dill, chopped

1. In a skillet, sauté carrots in oil for 2 minutes. Add water and brown rice syrup. Add several drops of tamari. Bring to boil, lower heat, and simmer, covered, 7 minutes, until carrots are tender.

2. Remove cover, raise flame, and allow remaining water to cook off. Sprinkle with lime juice and garnish with dill.

PER SERVING Calories: 55 | Fat: 1g | Sodium: 117mg | Carbohydrate: 11g | Fiber: 3g | Protein: 1g

Cutting Board Care

The cutting board should always be kept damp before cutting as a barrier against juices. Clean the cutting board with a damp cloth between cutting each vegetable. This preserves the polarity between vegetables, and keeps their energetic identities separate.

Baked Daikon, Turnip, and Rutabaga with Almond Kuzu Sauce

Baked root vegetables with kuzu sauce contain warming energy to balance cool autumn and winter weather. Pungent daikon and turnip strengthen lung and large intestine energy. Substitute various nut and seed butters for a different sauce.

INGREDIENTS | SERVES 4

Spring water, as needed
1 medium rutabaga, sliced ¼" thick
1 medium turnip, sliced ¼" thick
1 medium daikon, sliced ¼" thick
1 cup onion, sliced into half moons
1 teaspoon olive oil
Shoyu, to taste
1 teaspoon sweet white miso
2 teaspoons almond butter
2 teaspoons kuzu, dissolved in 1 cup water

Baking

Baking concentrates flavors in food while drying them out. Because protein and fat are brought to the surface, baked vegetables taste sweeter than those that are steamed. If you overuse this contracting cooking method, you may crave more oil and sweets for balance. Baking imparts warming energy to food and is more appropriate in cool weather.

1. Preheat oven to 350°F. Bring a pot of water to boil. Blanch rutabaga 7 minutes. Remove and layer on bottom of glass baking dish. Blanch turnip 5 minutes. Remove turnip and layer on top of rutabaga. Blanch daikon 5 minutes. Remove and layer on top of turnip.

2. Sauté onion in oil until translucent. Add shoyu, miso, and almond butter to kuzu water mixture. Add kuzu mixture to onions. Raise heat to high and stir until thickened.

3. Pour kuzu sauce over vegetables. Bake, uncovered, for 30 minutes.

PER SERVING Calories: 127 | Fat: 6g | Sodium: 81mg | Carbohydrate: 17g | Fiber: 4g | Protein: 3g

Boiled Salad with Carrots, Broccoli, and Cauliflower

Boiled salad is blanched vegetables that are crisp with upward rising energy. During blanching, vegetables turn bright colors, which are water soluble vitamins B and C coming to the surface. Vary seasonal vegetables and combinations daily. Serve with dressing or sauce.

INGREDIENTS | SERVES 3

Spring water, as needed
1 cup cauliflower florets
1 cup broccoli florets
1 cup carrots, cut into matchsticks
Umeboshi vinegar, optional

Blanching

Blanching means to boil vegetables separately until crisp. Because vegetables have different cooking rates, cooking each one separately prevents overcooking. This process also preserves their individual energy signatures. To retain flavor and preserve energy, begin with the mildest tasting, lightest colored vegetables and end with the strongest flavored ones.

1. Fill a saucepan with several inches of water. Bring to a boil.

2. Add cauliflower and boil 3 minutes. Remove cauliflower with a strainer and place in a mixing bowl. Reserve cooking water in saucepan.

3. Add broccoli and boil 2 minutes. Remove broccoli with a strainer and place broccoli in mixing bowl.

4. Add carrots and boil 1 minute. Remove carrots with a strainer and place carrots in mixing bowl.

5. Season with umeboshi vinegar, dressing, or sauce. Mix vegetables together.

PER SERVING Calories: 34 | Fat: 0g | Sodium: 48mg | Carbohydrate: 7g | Fiber: 2g | Protein: 2g

Fresh Shiitake, Onion, and Purple Cabbage Sauté

This dish contains settling soil energy, which is good for cool late summer weather.
Round vegetables, like onion and cabbage, support round middle organs.
Kuzu also has a warming effect and strengthens intestinal function.

INGREDIENTS | SERVES 2

1 cup onion, sliced into half moons
1 teaspoon sesame oil
1 cup fresh shiitake mushrooms, sliced
2 cups purple cabbage, sliced
½ cup spring water
Shoyu, to taste
1 teaspoon kuzu

1. In a skillet, sauté onion in oil for 3 minutes. Add shiitakes and sauté until cooked through.

2. Add cabbage and sauté until slightly wilted. Add ¼ cup water. Bring to boil, lower heat, and simmer, covered until cabbage is cooked.

3. Add shoyu, to taste. Dissolve kuzu in ¼ cup water. Add kuzu mixture to cabbage dish, stirring until thickened.

PER SERVING Calories: 107 | Fat: 2g | Sodium: 51mg | Carbohydrate: 18g | Fiber: 4g | Protein: 4g

Cruciferous Vegetables

Anticancer cruciferous vegetables are plants in the family *brassicaceae* (also called *cruciferae*), such as cabbage, broccoli, kale, and bok choy. Raw cruciferous vegetables can contain goitrogens, which are substances that can interfere with thyroid function in people with weakened thyroids. Cooking inactivates goitrogens and reduces their levels.

Purple Cabbage and Collards with Caramelized Onions

Caramelizing onions with a pinch of salt brings out their sweetness, which supports spleen, pancreas, and stomach energy. Caramelized red onions make a delicious garnish for greens, soups, fish, beans, pizza, salad, sandwiches, and vegetables.

INGREDIENTS | SERVES 6

1 medium red onion, sliced into half moons

1 tablespoon olive oil

⅛ teaspoon salt

2 tablespoons mirin

2 cups purple cabbage, chopped

2 cups collard greens, chopped

1 teaspoon thyme

¼ cup water

1 teaspoon lemon juice

¼ cup parsley

1. In a skillet, sauté onion in oil with a pinch of salt until onion is browned, about 10 minutes. Add mirin to skillet to deglaze pan. Allow mirin to simmer until almost evaporated. Remove onions to a bowl and set aside.

2. Add purple cabbage and collard greens. Sauté until greens begin to wilt. Add thyme and water and cover. Steam until tender, about 10 minutes.

3. Garnish with caramelized onions, lemon juice and parsley.

PER SERVING Calories: 50 | Fat: 2g | Sodium: 104mg | Carbohydrate: 7g | Fiber: 2g | Protein: 1g

Process of Cooking

Cooking methods affect the energy, flavor, and texture of food. Cooking is a controlled discharge of nutrients to the surface of food. Each cooking style has a unique quality and how vegetables are cut influences how they are cooked. A macrobiotic recipe maximizes delicious natural flavors without adding too much seasoning, while being energetically balanced.

Cauliflower, Portobello Mushroom, and Garbanzo Bean Stew

Downward settling soil energy in Garbanzo Bean Stew nourishes the spleen, pancreas, and stomach. Serve with pan fried mochi and mineral-rich foods (greens, sesame seeds, miso soup) to strengthen a weakened anemic condition, restoring blood and minerals.

INGREDIENTS | SERVES 8

1 medium onion, diced

2 medium portobello mushrooms, sliced

2 cloves garlic, crushed

2 teaspoons olive oil

1 head cauliflower, chopped

2 cups spring water, or broth

2 teaspoons kuzu

2 cups garbanzo beans, cooked

1 batch Baked Sweet Potato Sticks (page 235)

1 teaspoon salt

1 teaspoon lemon juice

½ cup parsley, chopped

1. In a Dutch oven, sauté onions, mushrooms, and garlic in oil until onions are translucent.

2. Add cauliflower and 1¾ cups water. Bring to boil, lower heat, and simmer, covered, for 10 minutes. Dissolve kuzu in ¼ cup cold water. Add cooked garbanzo beans, Baked Sweet Potato Sticks, salt, and kuzu mixture to stew. Cook for 5 minutes, stirring until thick.

3. Add lemon juice. Garnish with chopped parsley.

PER SERVING   Calories: 155 | Fat: 4g | Sodium: 356mg | Carbohydrate: 26g | Fiber: 7g | Protein: 7g

Cooking Factors

Both yin factors and yang factors are present during cooking. Yin factors are oil and water. Yang factors are salt, fire, pressure, and time. The seasoned chef knows when and how to use both yin and yang factors to create an energetically balanced dish. This is the art of macrobiotic cooking.

Carrot and Burdock Kimpira

Downward growing root vegetables carrot and burdock strengthen the intestines and counterbalance excess fire energy in the heart. Other vegetables to include are lotus root, beets, rutabaga, green beans, and sea vegetables. Oil sautéing puts a film around food, capturing its flavor and making it sweeter.

INGREDIENTS | SERVES 4

1 cup burdock, cut into thin matchsticks

1 teaspoon untoasted sesame oil

1 cup carrot, cut into thin matchsticks

Spring water, as needed

Shoyu, sea salt, or sweet white miso, to taste

Mirin or brown rice vinegar, to taste, optional

Kimpira

Kimpira (Japanese for "golden peace") is sautéed and simmered vegetables, usually carrots and burdock, cut into matchsticks. The effort of cutting vegetables into smaller pieces and sautéing puts active yang energy into this dish that is released in the body. This downward, contracting energy strengthens the large intestine and kidney.

1. In a skillet, sauté burdock in oil, about 2 minutes.

2. Spread burdock evenly over skillet and top with carrots. Do not stir. Add water to cover burdock only. Cover and cook over medium-low heat for about 10 minutes.

3. Season with shoyu, sea salt, or sweet white miso, cover, and cook a few more minutes. Season with mirin or brown rice vinegar, to taste (optional). Stir well before transferring to a serving platter.

PER SERVING   Calories: 4 | Fat: 1g | Sodium: 24mg | Carbohydrate: 8g | Fiber: 2g | Protein: 1g

Carrot, Cabbage, Burdock, and Daikon Nishime

Immune strengthening autumn nishime contains centering energy, which brings you back to balance. Kombu helps soften vegetables and adds minerals. You could season with umeboshi plum, ginger, sweet white miso, or shoyu, and thicken with kuzu or tahini.

INGREDIENTS | SERVES 4

1 stamp-sized piece kombu

½ cup spring water

1 cup daikon, cut into thick half moons

1 cup green cabbage, cut into 1" chunks

1 cup carrot, cut into 1" chunks

1 cup burdock, cut into ½" chunks

Pinch of salt

Shoyu, to taste

Nishime

Nishime (waterless cooking) is vegetable stew that is cooked in little water to concentrate flavors and nutrients. Vegetables are cut into large chunks and steamed slowly in ½" of water with kombu on the bottom of a heavy pot. This strengthening, centering cooking style nourishes the middle organs, which is good for hypoglycemia.

1. In a heavy pot, place kombu on bottom with water. Place vegetables in sections inside the pot. Add a pinch of salt over vegetables.

2. Bring to a boil, lower heat, and simmer, covered, for 15–20 minutes until soft.

3. Season with shoyu and simmer 3 more minutes.

4. Hold lid and handles with potholders. Lift covered pot and shake up and down to mix vegetables.

PER SERVING Calories: 45 | Fat: 0g | Sodium: 79mg | Carbohydrate: 10g | Fiber: 3g | Protein: 1g

Beet and Daikon Nishime with Fresh Dill

Nishime contains warming energy and is good for cool weather. Food is cooked in sections, which concentrates flavors and preserves their energetic identities. This is a variation that layers vegetables to blend energies and flavors together to create a sweet dish.

INGREDIENTS | SERVES 4

1 stamp-sized piece kombu
½ cup spring water
2 cups beets, sliced ½" thick
2 cups daikon, sliced ½" thick
Pinch salt
Shoyu, to taste
1 tablespoon fresh dill, chopped

Importance of Cutting

Cutting styles affect the energy, taste, and textures of food. Because cutting can either enhance or decrease nutrition, a particular cutting style must suit the dish. If vegetables are cut too small for a long-cooked dish, they may become over-cooked. Likewise, if vegetables are cut too large for a short cooked dish, they may be undercooked and indigestible.

1. In a wide pot, place kombu on bottom. Add water. Layer beets on bottom. Layer daikon on top of beets. Sprinkle a pinch of salt over daikon.

2. Bring to boil, lower heat, and simmer, covered, 20 minutes or until tender.

3. Season with shoyu, to taste. Simmer 3 more minutes.

4. Sprinkle dill over vegetables. Cover for 2 minutes. Serve.

PER SERVING   Calories: 38 | Fat: 0g | Sodium: 108mg | Carbohydrate: 8g | Fiber: 3g | Protein: 2g

Red Radish with Ume Kuzu Sauce

Roots and tops, such as radish with greens, energetically support both upper and lower regions of the body. Pungent red radish strengthens the large intestine, while bitter radish greens nourish heart function. For variety, use different kinds of roots, like daikon, carrot, and turnip, and their tops.

INGREDIENTS | SERVES 4

2 bunches whole red radish and tops

2 teaspoons umeboshi paste

¾ cups spring water

1 tablespoon kuzu

Role of Kuzu

Vegetable dishes may be thickened with kuzu water mixture at the end of cooking. Kuzu holds heat in the body and sustains this internal heat, which is especially beneficial in cool weather.

1. Place radishes, umeboshi paste, and ½ cup water in a saucepan. Bring to boil, lower heat, and simmer, covered, 2 minutes.

2. Add tops, cover, and continue to cook 2 minutes.

3. Dissolve kuzu in ¼ cup water. Add to radishes and tops. Cook 2 minutes, stirring until thick.

PER SERVING Calories: 14 | Fat: 0g | Sodium: 217mg | Carbohydrate: 4g | Fiber: 1g | Protein: 1g

CHAPTER 10

Gorgeous Greens

Blanched Collards with Ume Vinegar

Upward rising energy of blanched bitter greens supports liver and heart function.

INGREDIENTS | **SERVES 4**

1 bunch collards
6 cups spring water
Umeboshi vinegar, to taste

Greens

Because green leafy vegetables grow upward and outward, they support the upper part of the body, like the lungs and heart. This upward, rising, outward energy allows a closed heart to open itself to emotional connections and relationships. Greens can increase communication and social interaction, while nourishing the heart's capacity for joy.

1. Cut collards into 1" strips. Bring 6 cups spring water to boil. Drop collards into water. Cook collards 1–2 minutes. Drain.

2. Season with umeboshi vinegar, to taste.

PER SERVING Calories: 11 | Fat: 0g | Sodium: 7mg | Carbohydrate: 2g | Fiber: 1g | Protein: 1g

Bok Choy, Cilantro, and Shiitake Stir Fry

Asian stir fries often include savory sauces and vegetables that balance flavors (salty and sweet) and textures (crunchy and smooth). Because stir frying cooks food in a little oil over high heat, this summer cooking style seals in flavor as well as nutrition.

INGREDIENTS | SERVES 6

½ cup sea palm, soaked
1 cup shiitake mushrooms
½ medium onion, sliced into half-moons
2 cloves garlic, minced
1 tablespoon ginger, grated
2 tablespoons untoasted sesame oil
2 large carrots, cut into matchsticks
2 cups purple cabbage, shredded
1 head bok choy, thinly sliced
1 batch Almond Shiitake Miso Sauce (see below)
1 tablespoon sesame seeds, toasted
¼ cup cilantro, chopped

Almond Shiitake Miso Sauce

Almond Shiitake Miso Sauce flavors vegetables and noodles. Cook 2 large dried shiitake mushrooms in 3 cups water for 30 minutes. Strain. To broth, mix 2 tablespoons barley miso, 2 teaspoons mirin, 2 tablespoons almond butter, 2 teaspoons brown rice vinegar, 1 tablespoon brown rice syrup, and 2 tablespoons shoyu.

1. Drain sea palm. Slice sea palm into 2" strips. Remove stems from shiitakes and slice caps.

2. Sauté onions, garlic, and ginger in oil until onions are translucent. Add shiitake mushrooms and sauté until cooked. Add carrots and sauté 5 minutes. Add cabbage and white parts of bok choy and sauté 2 minutes. Add sea palm and Almond Shiitake Miso Sauce. Simmer 5 minutes.

3. Add green parts of bok choy. Simmer until greens are tender.

4. Garnish with sesame seeds and cilantro.

PER SERVING Calories: 171 | Fat: 9g | Sodium: 635mg | Carbohydrate: 18g | Fiber: 4g | Protein: 6g

Kale, Green Beans, and Carrots with Roasted Pumpkin Seeds

Full of summer energy, kale contains natural bitter flavor that supports heart function. Roasting pumpkin seeds also stimulates deficient heart energy.

INGREDIENTS | SERVES 4

1½ cups onion, sliced into half moons

2 cloves garlic, crushed

2 teaspoons olive oil

1½ cups carrots, cut into matchsticks

1½ cups green beans, diagonally sliced

¼ cup water

3 cups kale, chopped

1 batch Shoyu Lemon Tahini Sauce (see below)

½ cup pumpkin seeds, roasted

1. Sauté onions and garlic in oil until translucent.

2. Add carrots and green beans and sauté 1 minute. Add ¼ cup water. Bring to boil, lower heat, and simmer, covered, 6 minutes.

3. Add kale and continue to cook until kale is limp but still bright green, about 5 minutes. Add more water if needed.

4. Pour Shoyu Lemon Tahini Sauce on vegetables and mix. Sprinkle with roasted pumpkin seeds.

PER SERVING   Calories: 439 | Fat: 31g | Sodium: 550mg | Carbohydrate: 31g | Fiber: 9g | Protein: 19g

Shoyu Lemon Tahini Sauce

This sauce adds flavor to cooked beans, greens, and sautées. Heat ⅛ cup shoyu and ½ cup water for 2 minutes. Cool. Add juice of 1 lemon, ½ cup tahini, and ¼ cup scallions and purée. To make dip for sushi, heat ¼ cup shoyu and ¼ cup water for 2 minutes. Cool. Add ¼ teaspoon ginger or wasabi.

Dandelion Greens and Onion Sauté

Besides supporting heart function, bitter foods, like dandelion greens, naturally cleanse and detoxify the liver. Mineral-rich dandelion reduces inflammation of the liver and gallbladder, stimulates bile flow, and improves digestion.

INGREDIENTS | SERVES 4

1 bunch dandelion greens
1 cup onion, sliced into half moons
1 teaspoon olive oil
Shoyu, to taste

1. Cut dandelion greens into 1" strips. In a skillet, sauté onion in oil until translucent.

2. Add dandelion greens and sauté 1 minute.

3. Season greens with shoyu, to taste.

PER SERVING Calories: 51 | Fat: 2g | Sodium: 43mg | Carbohydrate: 9g | Fiber: 3g | Protein: 2g

Carrot Tops and Scallion Sauté

Bitter carrot tops nourish the heart's capacity for love and joy. Highly nutritious carrot greens are also rich in potassium, vitamin K, and cancer-fighting chlorophyll. Because they are diuretic, they can help treat kidney disease and edema.

INGREDIENTS | SERVES 2

1 bunch carrot tops
2–3 scallions, chopped
2 teaspoons olive oil
2 tablespoons spring water
Sweet brown rice vinegar, to taste

Cooking Bitter Greens

You can balance the strong bitter flavor of greens with sweet taste. Cook bitter greens, such as dandelion, turnip, radish, and carrot tops, with alliums, such as onion, shallots, leeks, or scallions. Alliums become sweet when cooked and contain settling energy to counterbalance expansive energy of bitter greens.

1. Chop carrot tops up to stems. In a skillet, sauté scallions in oil 1 minute.

2. Add carrot tops and sauté 1 minute. Add water. Bring to boil, lower heat, and simmer 2 minutes.

3. Season with sweet brown rice vinegar, to taste.

PER SERVING   Calories: 77 | Fat: 5g | Sodium: 53mg | Carbohydrate: 7g | Fiber: 3g | Protein: 3g

Braised Romaine Lettuce and Fennel

Mediterranean romaine lettuce and fennel are simmered in savory vegetable broth to add flavor. Rich in antioxidants, they are high in vitamin C, which is needed for proper immune system function. Crunchy fennel bulb also provides licorice flavor to this dish.

INGREDIENTS | **SERVES 4** |

1 large fennel bulb, cut into half moons
2 teaspoons olive oil
1 head romaine lettuce, cut into 2" strips
Salt, to taste
¼ cup vegetable broth

Braising

Braising is a method of cooking, often applied to meat, fish, or tempeh. These proteins are browned in fat or oil and simmered in a covered pot in a small amount of liquid (stock, water, wine). Vegetables can also be braised by searing in oil with a pinch of salt to lock in juices and then simmered in flavorful broth.

1. In a skillet, sauté fennel in oil for 5 minutes. Add lettuce, salt, and broth.

2. Bring to boil, lower heat, and simmer, covered, for 5 minutes. Serve.

PER SERVING Calories: 65 | Fat: 3g | Sodium: 102mg | Carbohydrate: 10g | Fiber: 5g | Protein: 3g

Steamed Baby Bok Choy with Shoyu

Baby bok choy is like getting two vegetables in one: crisp leafy greens and crunchy white stalks. Because stalks take longer to cook than green parts, they can be cooked separately. Tamari can be substituted for shoyu.

INGREDIENTS | SERVES 2

Water, as needed

3 cups baby bok choy, chopped

Shoyu, to taste

Steaming

Steaming cooks food, covered, with a small amount of water. Steaming energy is gathering, as water condenses in an enclosed pot. This conserves more minerals in food compared to boiling. While upward rising energy of boiling is appropriate for spring and summer, gathering steaming energy harmonizes with late summer and autumn.

1. Pour 1"–2" water into a pot with a lid. Insert a steamer basket in the pot.

2. Bring water to boil, covered. Add stalks to basket and cover. Steam 2–3 minutes.

3. Add green parts on top of stalks. Cover and steam 1 minute.

4. Season bok choy with shoyu, to taste.

PER SERVING Calories: 20 | Fat: 0g | Sodium: 98mg | Carbohydrate: 3g | Fiber: 2g | Protein: 2g

Mustard Greens and Lemon Sauté

Pungent mustard greens nourish lung function, benefiting asthma conditions and effects of long-time smoking. Health-promoting mustard greens have also been shown to protect against rheumatoid arthritis, cancer, memory loss, osteoporosis, and cardiovascular disorders.

INGREDIENTS | SERVES 4

1 bunch mustard greens, chopped

2 teaspoons untoasted sesame oil

2 tablespoons spring water

Lemon juice, to taste

¼ cup walnuts, toasted

1. In a skillet, sauté greens in oil for 2 minutes. Add water. Bring to boil, lower heat, and simmer, covered, 2 minutes.

2. Season with lemon juice. Chop walnuts and garnish over greens.

PER SERVING   Calories: 82 | Fat: 7g | Sodium: 14mg | Carbohydrate: 4g | Fiber: 2g | Protein: 3g

Short-Cooked Dishes

Short-cooked dishes add light, upward rising energy appropriate for warm weather. Light cooking styles, such as blanching, quick sauté, pressed salad, quick pickling, and raw, nourish the liver and heart. Include a short-cooked crispy dish, such as greens, daily, and vary the of greens used.

Sautéed Pea Shoots and Mung Bean Sprouts

Perfect for spring cooking, pea shoots and mung bean sprouts contain upward rising energy that nourishes liver function. Sprouting increases the amount of digestible vitamins A and C compared to no sprouting. The process of sprouting also converts starches to easily digestible simple sugars.

INGREDIENTS | SERVES 2

1 cup pea shoots, chopped

1 cup mung bean sprouts

2 teaspoons olive oil

2 tablespoons spring water

Shoyu, to taste

1. In a skillet, sauté pea shoots and mung bean sprouts in oil for 2 minutes. Add water. Bring to boil, lower heat, and simmer, covered, for 2 minutes.

2. Season with shoyu. Cook 2 more minutes. Serve.

PER SERVING Calories: 130 | Fat: 5g | Sodium: 15mg | Carbohydrate: 19g | Fiber: 1g | Protein: 7g

Steamed Watercress and Carrots

Steamed watercress and carrots contain downward gathering energy, which is appropriate for cool weather. An anticancer superfood, delicate watercress can reduce DNA damage to blood cells, and prevent the development of cancer.

INGREDIENTS | SERVES 4

Spring water, as needed

2 cups watercress, chopped

1 cup carrots, matchsticks

Umeboshi vinegar, to taste

Energy of Watercress

Each leafy green has signature essence which balances certain health conditions. Astringent watercress has the most contracted settling energy among greens. This energy counterbalances extreme upward rising (yin) chi in lymphoma and some breast cancer. Steaming watercress adds gathering energy. Season with shoyu or umeboshi vinegar at the end of cooking time.

1. In a saucepan, bring 1"–2" of water to a boil, and insert steamer basket. Add watercress and carrots. Cover and steam for 3 minutes.

2. Season with umeboshi vinegar, to taste.

PER SERVING Calories: 15 | Fat: 0g | Sodium: 29mg | Carbohydrate: 3g | Fiber: 1g | Protein: 1g

CHAPTER 11

Bodacious Beans

Black Soybeans with Chestnuts

Black soybeans are considered the crown prince of all soybeans. They increase blood circulation and water passage, counterbalance toxicity, and support kidney health. Rich in trace minerals, chestnuts are nutritionally similar to brown rice.

INGREDIENTS | SERVES 6

1 cup black soybeans, soaked in 4 cups water

¼ cup dried chestnuts, soaked

1 stamp-sized piece kombu, soaked

Shoyu, to taste

1. Place beans and soaking water in pressure cooker. Bring to boil. Skim off foam. Add chestnuts and kombu. Cover, bring to pressure, lower heat, and pressure cook for 50 minutes.

2. Season beans with shoyu, to taste.

PER SERVING Calories: 147 | Fat: 5g | Sodium: 17mg | Carbohydrate: 15g | Fiber: 7g | Protein: 12g

Doctrine of Signatures

A philosophy, called Doctrine of Signatures, states that a food that resembles an organ contains an energetic signature that nourishes that organ. As their name suggests, kidney beans strengthen kidneys and reproductive organs. Resembling kidneys in shape and having a split, beans benefit organs that come in halves, like kidneys.

Black Soybeans, Lotus Root, and Kabocha Squash

Nutritious black soybeans are rich in calcium, B vitamins, vitamin A, iron, phosphorus, magnesium, and zinc. Containing all essential amino acids, black soybeans are a complete protein food. Lotus root helps bind mucous in the lung and draw it out of the body.

INGREDIENTS | SERVES 6

1 cup black soybeans, soaked in 4 cups water

1 stamp-sized piece kombu, soaked

1 cup kabocha squash, cut into chunks

⅓ cup dried lotus root, soaked

Shoyu, to taste

Umeboshi paste, to taste

Toasted sesame oil, to taste

¼ cup parsley, chopped

1. Place beans and soaking water in a pressure cooker. Bring to boil. Skim off foam. Add kombu, squash, and dried lotus root. Cover, bring to pressure, lower heat, and pressure cook for 50 minutes.

2. Season beans with shoyu, to taste. Bring to boil, lower heat, and simmer, uncovered, for 2 minutes.

3. Season with umeboshi paste and toasted sesame oil, to taste. Garnish with parsley.

PER SERVING Calories: 148 | Fat: 4g | Sodium: 24mg | Carbohydrate: 15g | Fiber: 9g | Protein: 12g

Aduki Beans, Kombu, and Squash

Nourishing the middle organs and the kidney, this dish is good for diabetes and hypoglycemia. Experiment with various squashes, carrots, sautéed onion, and tempeh.

INGREDIENTS | SERVES 4

1 cup aduki beans, soaked in 4 cups water

1 stamp-sized piece kombu, soaked

1 cup kabocha squash, large chunks

Shoyu, to taste

½ cup mochi, grated, optional

¼ cup parsley, chopped

Preparing Beans for Cooking

Preparing beans for cooking makes them more digestible. First, remove stones from beans. Rinse beans under cool water, and soak 6–8 hours. Discard soaking water (except Hokkaido aduki and black soybean water, which is medicinal). Bring beans and water to boil, and remove foam. Then, cook beans with kombu to soften beans and balance oils.

1. In a heavy pot, add aduki beans and soaking water. Bring to boil and skim off foam. Add kombu and squash. Lower heat, and simmer, covered, 1½ hours. Add more water, if necessary, to cover beans.

2. Add shoyu and simmer another 15 minutes.

3. Stir grated mochi into hot beans to melt. Garnish with parsley.

PER SERVING   Calories: 175 | Fat: 0g | Sodium: 27mg | Carbohydrate: 34g | Fiber: 7g | Protein: 10g

Savory Navy Beans and Wild Mushrooms

Haricot beans were originally staple beans of the U.S. Navy in the early twentieth century. High in folate, magnesium, potassium, iron, and manganese, navy beans support cardiovascular health.

INGREDIENTS | SERVES 6

1 cup navy beans, soaked

4 cups spring water

1 clove, plus 2 tablespoons minced garlic

1 small carrot, diced

1 stalk celery, diced

1 stamp-sized piece kombu, soaked

2 cups onions, sliced into half moons

2 tablespoons sesame oil

8 ounces wild mushrooms, sliced

½ teaspoon dried tarragon

Shoyu, to taste

Lemon juice, to taste

¼ cup parsley, chopped

1. Rinse beans and place in a heavy stock pot. Add water, bring to boil, and remove foam. Add 1 clove garlic, carrot, celery, and kombu. Lower heat and cook until beans are tender, usually 60–90 minutes, or pressure cook for 25 minutes. Drain beans and set aside.

2. Sauté onions and 2 tablespoons minced garlic in oil in a large skillet over medium heat. Add wild mushrooms and tarragon and sauté until cooked through. Transfer onions and mushrooms to a bowl and set aside.

3. In a large bowl combine drained beans with the minced garlic, onions, and mushrooms. Season beans with shoyu, to taste. Add lemon juice, to taste, and garnish with parsley.

PER SERVING Calories: 179 | Fat: 3g | Sodium: 41mg | Carbohydrate: 30g | Fiber: 11g | Protein: 10g

Beautiful Black-Eyed Pea Burgers

Originating in Asia, warm weather black-eyed peas have upward rising and outward energy that supports liver and heart function. Rich in iron, calcium, and vitamin A, black-eyed peas add nutrition as well as strong meaty flavor to soups and vegan burgers.

INGREDIENTS | SERVES 6

1 cup black-eyed peas, soaked
Spring water, as needed
1 stamp-sized piece kombu, soaked
1 tablespoon umeboshi paste
2 medium scallions, chopped
¼ cup safflower oil

Protein Sources

Adequate dietary protein is necessary for normal muscle growth. Sources of protein in a macrobiotic diet are fish and beans. Fish is easily digestible, and contains less acidic protein that nourishes weak or deficient conditions. Beans are a nutritious, plant-based protein source: eat ½ to 1 cup beans daily, and up to 2 cups daily if you are protein deficient.

1. Rinse beans and place in a pressure cooker. Add enough water to cover beans by 1". Bring to boil. Skim off foam. Add kombu. Cover, bring to pressure, lower heat, and pressure cook for 20 minutes. (Or simmer on stove 1 hour.)

2. Mash beans. Season with umeboshi paste. Add scallions.

3. Form bean purée into 6–8 patties. Place in refrigerator to firm. In a skillet, pan fry patties in oil until browned on both sides.

PER SERVING Calories: 107 | Fat: 9g | Sodium: 187mg | Carbohydrate: 5g | Fiber: 2g | Protein: 1g

Garbanzo Beans in Mushroom Gravy

Chickpeas or garbanzo beans contain late summer energy, which supports digestion and nourishes the middle organs. Mushrooms contain spring energy, which strengthens liver function. Nutritious white mushrooms are rich in antioxidants and contain anticancer properties.

INGREDIENTS | SERVES 6

1½ cups garbanzo beans, soaked

Spring water, as needed, plus 2½ cups

1 stamp-sized piece kombu, soaked

1 medium onion, diced

1 teaspoon olive oil

12 white button mushrooms, sliced

2 tablespoons mirin (optional)

¼ cup shoyu

2 tablespoons kuzu

1. Drain beans and place in pressure cooker. Add enough water to cover beans by 1". Bring to boil and remove foam. Add kombu. Cover, bring to pressure, lower heat, and cook for 30 minutes.

2. Sauté onion in oil until translucent. Add mushrooms and sauté until cooked through. Add 2 cups water, mirin, and shoyu. Simmer 1 minute. Dissolve kuzu in ½ cup cold water. Add kuzu mixture to onions and simmer 2 minutes. Adjust seasonings to taste.

3. When beans are cooked, drain, and add to the mushroom gravy.

PER SERVING Calories: 210 | Fat: 4g | Sodium: 630mg | Carbohydrate: 37g | Fiber: 10g | Protein: 12g

Garlicky Garbanzo Beans

Garbanzo beans are used in late summer to strengthen the spleen, pancreas, and stomach. Pungent, antibacterial garlic was used traditionally to help thin the blood and enhance digestion. This dish makes a great snack or main dish, warm or cold.

INGREDIENTS | SERVES 6

1 cup garbanzo beans, soaked
Spring water, as needed
1 stamp-sized piece kombu, soaked
2 cloves garlic, roasted
¼ cup sesame seeds, toasted
1½ tablespoons umeboshi vinegar
¼ cup olive oil
2 medium scallions, chopped
¼ cup dill, chopped
Lemon juice, to taste

1. Drain garbanzo beans and place in pressure cooker. Add water to cover beans by 1". Bring to boil and remove foam. Add kombu and cover pressure cooker. Bring to pressure, lower heat, and pressure cook for 25 minutes. Drain beans.

2. Mince garlic. Grind toasted sesame seeds into powder. Season beans with umeboshi vinegar, olive oil, scallions, garlic, ground sesame seeds, dill, and lemon juice. Marinate beans overnight for best flavor before serving.

PER SERVING Calories: 240 | Fat: 14g | Sodium: 25mg | Carbohydrate: 23g | Fiber: 7g | Protein: 8g

Role of Cooking in Human Evolution

Cooking may have fueled human evolution. Cooking denatures proteins and breaks food down, making it more easily digestible. With nutrients more available, humans could expand their diets, freeing up energy from digestion to further development of the brain. Body size became larger, and teeth became smaller, as cooked roots required less chewing.

Baked Kidney Beans with Shiitake, Burdock, and Onion Gravy

Nutritious kidney beans are rich in folate and magnesium, which have been associated with decreased risk of heart attack. Iron-rich kidney beans are good for building blood, especially for children, adolescents, and women who are pregnant, lactating, or menstruating.

NGREDIENTS | SERVES 6

1 cup kidney beans, soaked

Spring water, as needed, plus 2¼ cups

1 stamp-sized piece kombu

1 medium burdock, sliced into matchsticks

2 teaspoons olive oil

1 medium onion, sliced into half moons

1 cup shiitake mushrooms, sliced

1 tablespoon kuzu

Shoyu, to taste

Cooking Kidney Beans

Delicious in chili, salad, soup, and grain dishes, kidney beans become soft and creamy when pressure cooked for 25 minutes. An alternative is to cook kidney beans using the "crock pot" method. Bring beans to boil, place a flame deflector under the pot, lower heat, and simmer on pilot light overnight.

1. Drain beans and place in pressure cooker. Add enough water to cover beans by 1". Bring to a boil and remove foam. Add kombu and cover pressure cooker. Bring to pressure, lower heat, and pressure cook for 25 minutes. Drain beans, saving bean liquid. Pour beans into baking pan.

2. In a skillet, sauté burdock in oil for 2 minutes. Add onion and sauté until translucent. Add shiitakes and sauté until cooked through. Add 1¼ cups water. Bring to a boil, lower heat, and simmer, covered, for 10 minutes.

3. Dissolve kuzu in 1 cup water or bean liquid. Add kuzu mixture to vegetables. Raise heat to high and stir until think. Season with shoyu, to taste.

4. Preheat oven to 350°F. Pour gravy over beans and bake for 30 minutes.

PER SERVING Calories: 150 | Fat: 2g | Sodium: 29mg | Carbohydrate: 27g | Fiber: 9g | Protein: 8g

Savory French Green Lentils

Tiny, delicate French green lentils are grown in the Puy region in the Auvergne area of France. Their nutty flavor comes from the mineral-rich volcanic soil in which they are grown. Because they have less starch than other lentils, they are ideal for salads. Ingredients can include cooked beets and beet greens.

INGREDIENTS | SERVES 6

1 cup French green lentils, soaked

Spring water, as needed

1 stamp-sized piece kombu, soaked

1 cup onion, diced

1 medium carrot, diced

1 teaspoon untoasted sesame oil

Toasted sesame oil, to taste

Umeboshi vinegar, to taste

Lemon juice, to taste

¼ cup parsley, chopped

1. Drain lentils. Place lentils in a saucepan and cover with water. Bring to boil and remove foam. Add kombu, lower heat, and simmer for 25–30 minutes or until tender, adding more water if needed. Drain.

2. In a skillet, sauté onion and carrot in untoasted sesame oil until tender. Mix carrot and onion with lentils.

2. Season lentils and vegetables with toasted sesame oil, umeboshi vinegar, and lemon juice to taste.

3. Garnish with parsley.

PER SERVING Calories: 136 | Fat: 3g | Sodium: 28mg | Carbohydrate: 22g | Fiber: 6g | Protein: 7g

Cooking with Salt Sources

Because salt sources (sea salt, tamari, shoyu, miso) contain contracting yang energy, cooking them into food (3–4 minutes) balances energies in a dish. If you need more salt, heat it in a little water until dissolved (5–7 minutes), as raw salt is difficult to digest. Cook shoyu and water (2–3 minutes), instead of using raw shoyu, or add umeboshi vinegar instead.

Luscious Lima Beans and Corn

Succotash is a Southern dish traditionally made with lima beans and dried corn that is often served at Thanksgiving. Green beans or kidney beans can be used in place of lima beans. Vegetables like sun-dried tomatoes, squash, edamame, onions, and peas can be included.

INGREDIENTS | SERVES 6

1 cup lima beans, soaked

Spring water, as needed

1 stamp-sized piece kombu, soaked

3 cups fresh corn kernels

1 teaspoon olive oil

2 teaspoons sweet white miso

¼ cup chives, chopped

1. Drain beans. Place beans in a saucepan and cover with water by 1". Bring to boil and remove foam. Add kombu, lower heat, and simmer for 1½ hours or until tender, adding more water if needed.

2. Add corn, olive oil, and sweet white miso. Simmer for 5 minutes.

3. Garnish with chives.

PER SERVING Calories: 184 | Fat: 3g | Sodium: 68mg | Carbohydrate: 34g | Fiber: 8g | Protein: 9g

Neptune's Sea Vegetables

Vegan Hijiki Caviar

Downward gathering energy of hijiki stabilizes excess heart energy, which can manifest as mental illness. Mineral-rich hijiki also detoxifies body tissues, purifies blood, reduces blood pressure, and has a strengthening effect on the intestines.

INGREDIENTS | SERVES 4

½ cup hijiki, soaked 30 minutes

Apple juice to cover hijiki

2 cloves garlic, minced

2 shallots, minced

2 tablespoons sesame oil

2 tablespoons shoyu

Brown rice vinegar, to taste

1 tablespoon ginger, grated and juiced

18 pieces brown rice crackers

Toasted sesame seeds, optional

Fresh chives or dill sprigs, optional

Orange zest, optional

Hijiki: Nature's Miracle Worker

Hijiki helps bind and draw out toxins in the body. Hijiki contains valuable nutrients and compounds called arsenosugars. Arsenosugars metabolize, break down, and eliminate toxins, like inorganic arsenic, in the body. (Organic arsenic readily decomposes into sugar.) Because of its high mineral content, hijiki needs to be presoaked.and the soaking water discarded. Visit edenfoods.com to learn more: *www.edenfoods.com/articles/view.php?articles_id=79.*

1. Remove hijiki from water and place in a saucepan. Add apple juice to cover hijiki. Bring to boil, lower heat, and simmer, covered, for 20 minutes.

2. Remove hijiki from apple juice. In a skillet, sauté garlic and shallots in sesame oil until translucent. Add hijiki and sauté for 4 minutes. Add shoyu and cook until all liquid is evaporated.

3. Remove hijiki to cutting board and finely chop.

4. Season with brown rice vinegar and ginger juice if needed.

5. Serve on brown rice crackers or sliced and toasted whole wheat toast topped with toasted sesame seeds, chives, dill, or orange zest.

PER SERVING Calories: 138 | Fat: 8g | Sodium: 621mg | Carbohydrate: 14g | Fiber: 1g | Protein: 3g

Hijiki, Squash, and Onion Sauté

Sautéing calcium-rich hijiki in oil helps the body absorb minerals. This counterbalances acid blood, which contributes to osteoporosis and hair loss. This sauté is also good for nourishing diabetes and anemia. Cooking in cast iron adds strengthening energy to this dish.

INGREDIENTS | SERVES 6

1 cup onions, cut into half moons

1 teaspoon sesame oil

½ cup hijiki, soaked 30 minutes

Water to cover hijiki

1 cup winter squash, peeled and cubed

1 carrot, cut into matchsticks

Shoyu, to taste

Ginger juice or brown rice vinegar, to taste (optional)

2 tablespoons parsley, for garnish

1 tablespoon sesame seeds, toasted

Balancing Sea Vegetables

Balance yang sea vegetables with yin ingredients, such as sweet vegetables, protein (tempeh, dried tofu), greens, tahini, seeds, nuts, or citrus juice. Adding sweet and sour tastes to sea vegetable dishes helps you digest their minerals. Cook hijiki in apple juice instead of water. Longtime cooking or soaking also improves hijiki's digestibility.

1. In a skillet, sauté onions in oil until translucent, about 5–7 minutes.

2. Cut hijiki into 1½"-long pieces. Add hijiki and sauté 5 more minutes. Add water to cover hijiki. Bring to boil, lower heat, and simmer, covered, for 10 minutes.

3. Add squash, cover, and cook for 10 minutes.

4. Add carrots, cover, and cook 5 more minutes. Remove cover, season with shoyu and ginger juice, and cook until liquid has evaporated.

5. Garnish with parsley and toasted sesame seeds.

PER SERVING Calories: 38 | Fat: 2g | Sodium: 36mg | Carbohydrate: 6g | Fiber: 1g | Protein: 1g

Arame with Carrots, Beets, and Onions

Arame strengthens the middle organs and female reproductive system. This long-growing sea vegetable contains mannitol (non-caloric sugar), which stabilizes blood pressure and blood sugar levels. Other vegetables you can include are green beans, corn, and edamame.

INGREDIENTS | SERVES 4

1 medium red onion, cut into half moons

1 teaspoon sesame oil

1 cup arame, rinsed

½ cup beets, cut into matchsticks

½ cup carrots, cut into matchsticks

Spring water, as needed

1½ tablespoons tamari, or to taste

Brown rice vinegar, to taste

1 tablespoon fresh dill, chopped

Layering Sea Vegetables

When cooking sea vegetables, the energy of a dish depends on how food is layered. Sea vegetables layered on the bottom absorb flavors of other vegetables, becoming sweeter and milder. Sea vegetables layered on top, however, are drier and retain their own essence, becoming stronger in flavor.

1. In a skillet, sauté onion in oil until translucent. Layer arame on top of onions, beets on top of arame, and carrots on top of beets. Add water halfway up arame layer. Bring to boil, lower heat, and simmer 20 minutes.

2. Season with tamari, stir, and continue to cook, uncovered, until liquid has evaporated.

3. Season to taste with brown rice vinegar. Garnish with dill. Cover for 2 minutes. Serve.

PER SERVING Calories: 54 | Fat: 1g | Sodium: 463mg | Carbohydrate: 10g | Fiber: 5g | Protein: 9g

Tempeh with Arame, Shiitake, and Onion Gravy

Served with polenta, arame helps discharge soft dairy, which accumulates in the upper region of the body. Tahini, which has a creamy consistency, can be added to gravy to satisfy ice cream and soft dairy cravings.

INGREDIENTS | SERVES 4

6 medium dried shiitake mushrooms, soaked in 2 cups spring water

⅓ cup onion, finely diced

2 cloves garlic, minced

2 teaspoons sesame oil

8 ounces tempeh, cut into 1" cubes

¼ cup arame, rinsed

1½ tablespoons shoyu

2 tablespoons kuzu

¼ cup cold spring water

1. Remove mushroom stems and save soaking water. Slice caps and set aside.

2. In a skillet, sauté onion and garlic in oil until translucent. Add tempeh, arame, mushroom soaking liquid, shoyu, and shiitake mushrooms. Bring to a boil, lower heat, and simmer, covered, for 20 minutes.

3. Dissolve kuzu in ¼ cup cold water. Add kuzu water mixture to gravy. Bring to boil, lower heat, and stir until mixture thickens. Add additional shoyu if needed, to taste.

PER SERVING   Calories: 158 | Fat: 8g | Sodium: 362mg | Carbohydrate: 16g | Fiber: 2g | Protein: 13g

Cooking Arame

Because it has been presoaked and pre-cooked, rinse dried arame, instead of soaking, to preserve mineral content. When you are ready to cook, cover arame with water in a bowl. Give arame a shake to loosen tiny shells and sand, and transfer arame into another bowl. Now it is ready to use in vegetable dishes.

Fried Rice with Wild Nori

Iron- and vitamin-rich wild Atlantic nori (laver) is a cousin of Japanese nori. Roasted laver is delicious as a snack, included in trail mix, or crumbled into soups, salads, or popcorn. Add various vegetables in fried rice, such as corn, peas, cabbage, and mushrooms.

INGREDIENTS | SERVES 6

½ cup wild nori
1 cup red onion, diced
2 cloves garlic, crushed
1 tablespoon olive oil
½ teaspoon sesame oil
1 medium carrot, cut into matchsticks
½ cup celery, diced
½ cup broccoli, chopped
3 cups cooked brown rice
4 tablespoons water
3 tablespoons shoyu
2 medium scallions, sliced
Gomashio, to taste

1. Toast wild nori in the oven at 300°F for 5–8 minutes, turning occasionally, until crisp. Crumble or cut into flakes.

2. In a wok or heavy skillet, sauté onion and garlic in olive and sesame oil for 5–7 minutes. Add carrots and celery and sauté for 5 minutes. Add broccoli and sauté 5 minutes more. Add cooked rice, water, and shoyu and stir for 2 minutes. Taste and adjust seasonings. Add nori and stir.

3. Garnish with scallions and gomashio.

PER SERVING Calories: 162 | Fat: 4g | Sodium: 525mg | Carbohydrate: 29g | Fiber: 3g | Protein: 4g

Nori

Delicately growing nori nourishes the circulatory system, reduces blood pressure, and helps prevent hardening of the arteries. Nori enriches and cleanses the blood, discharging toxins. Because it is antibiotic and helps align tissues for healing, it can be used at home and while traveling as first aid for small cuts.

Root Vegetables and Sea Palm

Nourishing the middle organs, sea palm and sweet root vegetables provide a relaxing effect. Downward gathering energy of carrot and burdock roots help ground the lower half of the body. Experiment with various root vegetables, or add tempeh or mushrooms for a heartier dish.

INGREDIENTS | SERVES 6

1 medium burdock root, cut into matchsticks

2 teaspoons sesame oil, toasted

1 medium onion, sliced into half moons

1 medium carrot, cut into matchsticks

½ cup sea palm, soaked in 1½ cups water

1 tablespoon shoyu

2 tablespoons sesame seeds, toasted

1 tablespoon fresh dill, chopped

1. Sauté burdock in sesame oil for 2 minutes. Add onion and sauté until onion is translucent. Add carrot and sauté 1–2 minutes.

2. Add 1½ cups of sea palm soaking water and layer sea palm on top of vegetables. Add shoyu. Cover and simmer for 20 minutes. Remove cover and allow remaining liquid to evaporate.

3. Toss with sesame seeds. Garnish with dill. Cover for 2 minutes. Serve.

PER SERVING Calories: 59 | Fat: 2g | Sodium: 218mg | Carbohydrate: 9g | Fiber: 2g | Protein: 2g

Cooking with Sea Palm

Like arame, sea palm is used in salads and vegetable dishes. Soak sea palm for a couple of hours to rehydrate and save its nutritious soaking water to use as broth. Cook sea palm with sweet vegetables, like winter squash, onion, carrot, corn, beet, and cabbage. Using oil in sautés helps minerals to be absorbed in the body.

Land and Sea Vegetable Salad

Land and sea merge together into this immune-strengthening, mineral-rich salad. Soaked wakame, couscous, chickpeas, and corn can be included. Orange Sesame Dressing (page 193) can be used as seasoning in place of shoyu and sweet brown rice vinegar.

INGREDIENTS | SERVES 4

½ cup snow pea pods

Spring water, as needed

Pinch sea salt

½ cup carrots, cut into matchsticks

½ cup sea palm, soaked

½ cup sea whip fronds, soaked

4 tablespoons sweet brown rice vinegar

1 tablespoon shoyu

1 tablespoon toasted sesame oil

Toasted walnuts, chopped, optional

Orange zest, optional

1. Remove ends and strings from snow pea pods. Bring one pot of water to boil and add a pinch of sea salt. Boil carrots for 2–3 minutes and remove with a slotted spoon. Boil pea pods 1–2 minutes and remove with a slotted spoon. Chop sea vegetables to desired length. Place all vegetables and sea vegetables in a mixing bowl.

2. Add sweet brown rice vinegar, shoyu, and sesame oil and stir. Garnish with toasted chopped walnuts and orange zest.

PER SERVING   Calories: 56 | Fat: 4g | Sodium: 438mg | Carbohydrate: 5g | Fiber: 1g | Protein: 2g

Bladderwrack Vegetable Soup

Bladderwrack is bladder-shaped form of kelp used to treat bladder infections. Rich in iodine, it stimulates thyroid function and weight loss by boosting metabolism. Bladderwrack also helps relieve rheumatoid arthritis and inflammation.

INGREDIENTS | SERVES 2

1½ large shiitake mushrooms, sliced

1 tablespoon toasted sesame oil

2½ cups spring water

½ medium carrot, diced

½ ounce bladderwrack, soaked

½ package udon noodles, cooked

1 teaspoon barley miso

1 teaspoon shoyu

2 teaspoons lemon juice

2 tablespoons scallions, chopped

1. In a soup pot, sauté shiitakes in oil until cooked through. Add water, carrots, and bladderwrack. Bring to boil, lower heat, and simmer, covered for 15 minutes.

2. Add cooked udon noodles, miso, and shoyu and cook for 2 minutes.

3. Season with lemon juice. Garnish with scallions.

PER SERVING Calories: 277 | Fat: 9g | Sodium: 950mg | Carbohydrate: 43g | Fiber: 4g | Protein: 9g

Energy of Sea Vegetables

Rich in minerals, sea vegetables are like rocks, which have the ability to retain "ancient memory." Eating sea vegetables helps you connect with spirit and the memory of eternal present, being here in this moment. Strengthening the kidney and bladder, sea vegetables enhance courage and standing in your truth.

Harvest Stew with Irish Moss

High in life-enhancing vitamins and minerals, Irish moss (carrageen moss) nourishes the skin and strengthens the lung and respiratory system. It is used to treat urinary tract infections, ulcers, cancer, thyroid problems, and radiation poisoning.

INGREDIENTS | SERVES 6

1½ medium onions, sliced into half moons

2 teaspoons sesame oil

8 ounces shiitake mushrooms, sliced

3 cups butternut squash, peeled

5 cups spring water

1½ cups daikon, cut into 1" chunks

1½ large carrots, cut into 1" chunks

¾ cup parsnip, cut into 1" chunks

1½ stalks celery, diced

¼ cup Irish moss, soaked

Sea salt, to taste

Lemon juice, to taste

¼ cup parsley, chopped

1. In a skillet, sauté onions in oil until translucent. Add shiitake mushrooms and sauté until cooked through.

2. Cut squash into chunks. In a soup pot add water, daikon, squash, carrot, and parsnip. Bring to boil, lower heat, and simmer, covered, for 20 minutes.

3. Add onions, shiitake mushrooms, and celery. Simmer 20 minutes more.

4. Rinse Irish moss and add to stew. Add sea salt, to taste. Simmer for 5 minutes or until thick.

5. Stir well to dissolve squash into a creamy, thick sauce. Season with lemon juice. Garnish with parsley.

PER SERVING Calories: 121 | Fat: 2g | Sodium: 283mg | Carbohydrate: 19g | Fiber: 4g | Protein: 9g |

Kelp Noodle Salad

Rich sources of iodine and trace minerals, kelp noodles are a nutritious addition to broths, sautés, salads, and vegetable spring rolls. Season kelp noodles with any dressing or sauce, or use in place of pasta, cellophane noodles (Korean bean threads), or rice vermicelli.

INGREDIENTS | SERVES 4

6 ounces kelp noodles, rinsed
¼ cup cucumber, thinly sliced
4 cups spring water
¼ cup carrots, cut into matchsticks
2 tablespoons sweet white miso
2 tablespoons brown rice syrup
1 tablespoon stone ground mustard
Sesame oil, to taste

1. In a bowl, add kelp noodles and cucumber. Bring 4 cups spring water to boil. Add carrots and blanch 1 minute. Remove and add to kelp noodles and cucumber.

2. Mix together sweet white miso, brown rice syrup, stone ground mustard, and sesame oil. Combine with kelp noodles, carrot, and cucumber.

PER SERVING Calories: 62 | Fat: 0g | Sodium: 234mg | Carbohydrate: 12g | Fiber: 1g | Protein: 1g

CHAPTER 13

Strengthening Soups

Basic Miso Soup

A mineral-rich blood purifier, this soup counterbalances excess rising energy from overconsumption of sugar. Vary the kinds of seasonal vegetables and greens daily. You can even add sautéed onions, baked mochi croutons, grains, beans, or noodles.

INGREDIENTS | SERVES 4

2 small dried shiitake mushrooms, soaked in 4 cups water

1 piece wakame, 3" long, soaked

½ cup carrot, diced

½ cup fresh peas

½ cup arugula, chopped

4 teaspoons barley miso

Lemon juice, to taste

Energy of Miso

Like fine wine, miso has many flavors, aromas, colors, and textures. Three-year-old dark miso (barley or brown rice) is more yang and strengthening than six-month-old white miso (chickpea), which is sweeter and more yin. Because it absorbs energetic signatures of all four seasons, eating dark miso brings you in touch with the natural rhythms within you.

1. Remove stems from mushrooms. Slice mushroom caps. Slice wakame into thin strips. In a medium saucepan, bring mushroom soaking water to boil. Add wakame, mushroom caps, and carrot. Lower heat, and simmer, covered, for 5 minutes.

2. Add fresh peas and simmer 5 more minutes. Add arugula and simmer for 15 seconds.

3. Remove a little broth and purée with miso in a suribachi bowl.

4. Pour miso purée into soup. Simmer for 2 minutes. Add lemon juice to taste.

PER SERVING Calories: 29 | Fat: 0g | Sodium: 217mg | Carbohydrate: 5g | Fiber: 1g | Protein: 2g

Clear Broth with Sweet White Miso

This strengthening broth is nourishing by itself or with cooked noodles, pressure cooked chickpeas, and vegetables. Any light-colored vegetable can create a clear broth: daikon, scallions, turnip, cabbage hearts, white part of leeks, yellow squash, celery, cauliflower, corn, and shallots.

INGREDIENTS | SERVES 5

1 stamp-sized piece kombu, soaked
½ medium onion, sliced
1 cup bok choy, white part only
4 cups spring water
4 teaspoons sweet white miso
Sea salt, to taste
½ sheet nori
½ scallion, sliced

Vegetable Broth

Instead of using whole vegetables, save vegetable scraps, shiitake stems, and lemon rinds to make broth. Cover vegetables with water, bring to boil, lower heat, and simmer 20 minutes, covered. Strain out scraps and use broth for soups or other vegetable dishes.

1. Place kombu, onion, and bok choy in a soup pot and add water.

2. Bring to a boil, lower heat, and simmer for 10 minutes, covered. Strain vegetables.

3. Purée miso with a little broth and add purée to rest of broth. Season with sea salt. Simmer for 3 minutes.

4. Slice nori into ½" × 3" long strips. Garnish broth with nori and scallions.

PER SERVING Calories: 16 | Fat: 0g | Sodium: 120mg | Carbohydrate: 3g | Fiber: 1g | Protein: 1g

Passion Beet Borscht

This is a creamy version of the classic Russian-style soup. Beets are nutrition-packed elixirs of life, chock full of anti-aging, immune-boosting nutrient compounds. Beet juice is also helpful for relaxing an overly contracted health condition.

INGREDIENTS | SERVES 4

2 cups beets, diced

5 cups spring water

1 medium carrot, diced

1 medium parsnip, diced

1 medium onion, diced

1½ teaspoons caraway seeds

½ cup red cabbage, chopped

1 teaspoon sesame oil

4 teaspoons sweet white miso

Lemon juice, to taste

¼ cup fresh dill, chopped

Cooking with Water

The energy of a dish depends on how much water you add and when you add it. Adding water at the beginning of cooking dilutes flavors and makes a weaker dish. To make flavors stronger and more concentrated, add less water at the beginning and then add more water later (this does not dissolve the first effect).

1. In a saucepan, add beets in water. Bring to boil, cover, and simmer for about 15 minutes.

2. Add carrot and parsnip and continue to cook over medium heat until vegetables are tender, about 15 minutes.

3. In a skillet, sauté onions with caraway seeds and cabbage in oil until soft. Add onions and cabbage to the soup.

4. Purée miso in a little cooking liquid. Add miso purée to soup and simmer for 3 more minutes.

5. Purée soup in a blender until creamy. Add lemon juice to taste. Garnish with freshly chopped dill.

PER SERVING Calories: 68 | Fat: 1g | Sodium: 148mg | Carbohydrate: 13g | Fiber: 3g | Protein: 2g

Kabocha Squash and Parsnip Purée

Enjoy this warming soup when late summer weather becomes cool. Sweet creamy squash soup is perfect for nourishing diabetes. Different versions of this soup can be made using various winter squash: butternut, buttercup, acorn, or carnival. Peel squash skins if they are tough.

INGREDIENTS | SERVES 4

1 medium onion, diced

1 clove garlic, crushed

1 teaspoon sesame oil

4 cups spring water

3 cups kabocha squash, cubed

1 cup parsnips, diced

1 piece wakame, 3" long, soaked

4 teaspoons sweet white miso

Shoyu, to taste

Lemon juice, to taste

¼ cup fresh dill, chopped

1. In a soup pot, sauté onion and garlic in oil over medium heat.

2. Add water, squash, parsnips, and wakame. Bring to boil, and simmer, covered, for 30 minutes.

3. Season with sweet white miso. Purée in a food mill or blender. Return soup to pot. Season with shoyu, to taste, and simmer, covered, 3 minutes.

4. Add lemon juice, to taste. Garnish with chopped dill.

PER SERVING   Calories: 88 | Fat: 1g | Sodium: 141mg | Carbohydrate: 18g | Fiber: 3g | Protein: 2g

Role of Garnish

Garnish helps balance a dish. Not only does it add another flavor and other nutritional factors, it balances the energy of a dish. Light green garnish provides an upward rising effect that balances heavy, salty, gathering energy. Some garnishes are scallions, parsley, watercress, chives, arugula, grated carrots, grated ginger, lemon zest, dill, cilantro, and nori.

Turkish Lentil Soup

Lentils support upward rising energy of the liver. Luscious and mouthwatering, this soup is quick cooking and can be eaten cool as a side dish on a hot day. Seasoning soup with lemon juice or brown rice vinegar gives it a lift.

INGREDIENTS | SERVES 4

¼ cup onion, diced

1 clove garlic, crushed

1 teaspoon sesame oil

½ teaspoon dried sage

½ teaspoon cumin powder

½ teaspoon dried thyme

1 piece wakame, 3" long, soaked

4 cups spring water

1 medium carrot, diced

1 cup red lentils

Shoyu, to taste

Lemon juice, to taste

¼ cup scallions, chopped

Hearty Soup: The Main Attraction

A hearty soup that is concentrated in flavor can serve as the main dish. If the soup is strong and thick like stew, design a lighter meal (sushi, lentil soup, and greens) around the soup. Likewise, a lighter meal, such as a quick lunch, can include a stronger soup or stew as the main course.

1. In a soup pan, sauté onion and garlic in oil with sage, cumin, and thyme until tender.

2. Slice wakame into thin strips. Add water, wakame, carrot, and lentils. Bring to a boil, remove foam, lower heat, and simmer until lentils are tender, about 40 minutes.

3. Add shoyu, to taste, and simmer for 5 more minutes.

4. Place all but 1 cup soup in a food processor or blender and blend briefly. Return blended soup to the pot with the reserved cup of soup.

5. Season to taste with more shoyu and lemon juice. Garnish with scallions.

PER SERVING Calories: 196 | Fat: 2g | Sodium: 44mg | Carbohydrate: 32g | Fiber: 8g | Protein: 14g

Vegan Clam Soup

Reminiscent of New England clam chowder, this soup includes clam-flavored oyster mushrooms and health-promoting shiitake mushrooms. Shiitakes support liver function and help dissolve animal fat in the body. Coconut milk can be added in place of almond milk for richer consistency.

INGREDIENTS | SERVES 4

1 medium onion, diced
2 cloves garlic, crushed
1 teaspoon olive oil
6 ounces oyster mushrooms, sliced
2 large fresh shiitake mushrooms
4 cups vegetable broth
½ stalk celery, diced
½ teaspoon dried tarragon
1 medium bay leaf
Sea salt, to taste
Shoyu, to taste
1 cup Almond Milk (page 225)
¼ cup parsley, chopped

1. In a large soup pot, sauté onions and garlic in oil until soft. Add mushrooms and sauté until cooked, about 8 minutes.

2. Add broth, celery, tarragon, and bay leaf. Bring to boil, lower heat, and simmer, covered, until vegetables are soft, about 10 minutes.

3. Season with salt and shoyu. Add almond milk. Simmer, covered, for 3 minutes. Remove half of the soup and purée in blender. Return puréed soup to pot.

4. Garnish with parsley.

PER SERVING Calories: 121 | Fat: 7g | Sodium: 961mg | Carbohydrate: 12g | Fiber: 2g | Protein: 4g

The Role of Salt

Adding salt during cooking causes vegetables to contract. If you want to conserve the flavor of vegetables, add salt seasonings at the beginning of cooking. However, if you want vegetables to flavor the broth, add salt, miso, tamari, shoyu, or umeboshi plum at the end of cooking.

Lovely Lentil Soup with Greens

Beauty is a reflection of what goes in your body as well as what goes on it. Rich in fiber, lentils stabilize blood sugar levels, lower cholesterol, and improve cardiovascular health. These health benefits create radiant beauty from the inside out.

INGREDIENTS | SERVES 5

1 cup lentils, soaked

1 cup onion, diced

1 teaspoon sesame oil

2 cloves garlic, crushed

1 teaspoon cumin

4–5 cups spring water

½ cup winter squash

1 piece wakame, 3" long, soaked

1 medium bay leaf

¼ cup celery, diced

½ cup carrot, diced

1½ tablespoon sweet white miso

1 cup kale or collards, chopped into bite-sized pieces

Lemon juice, to taste

Adjusting Cooking for Cool Weather

Adjust your cooking to create hearty (yang) meals in cool (yin) weather. To make a dish more yang, use cooking methods that add warming energy and concentrate flavors, such as pressure cooking, adding more salt, increasing cooking time, cutting vegetables into bigger chunks, using a heavy pot, and using less water.

1. Soak lentils overnight and drain. In a stockpot, sauté onion in oil until translucent. Add garlic and cumin and cook for 1 minute.

2. Add lentils and water, bring to a boil, and skim off the foam.

3. Peel squash and cut into ½" chunks. Slice wakame into thin strips. Add squash, wakame, bay leaf, and remaining vegetables except greens to pot. Bring to boil, lower heat, and simmer until lentils are soft, about 45 minutes.

4. Purée miso with a little cooking liquid. Add miso purée to soup.

5. Add greens and simmer, covered, for 5 minutes. Season with lemon juice.

PER SERVING Calories: 186 | Fat: 2g | Sodium: 144mg | Carbohydrate: 32g | Fiber: 13g | Protein: 11g

Garden Greens Soup with Garbanzos

Bring the garden into the kitchen with wild vegetables that imbibe the energy of nature. When you eat fresh-picked food, you absorb this living energy—this is soul food. Garbanzos contain late summer energy and support spleen, pancreas, and stomach function.

INGREDIENTS | SERVES 6

½ cup dried garbanzo beans, soaked

Water, as needed to cover beans, plus 5 cups

1 stamp-sized piece kombu

½ medium yellow onion, diced

1 clove garlic, minced

1 teaspoon sesame oil

3 ounces fresh shiitake mushrooms, sliced

1 medium bay leaf

½ teaspoon dried thyme

1½ tablespoons sweet white miso

1 cup kale or collards, chopped into bite-sized pieces

Lemon juice, to taste

Choose Your Destiny

Because you control what energy goes into your body, you choose your destiny whenever you decide what to cook. For example, the more an onion cooks, the sweeter it becomes. So, to add the sweetness of an onion to a dish, add the onion first. However, to add the pungent flavor of an onion, add the onion last.

1. Drain garbanzos and place them in a medium saucepan. Add water to cover and bring to boil. Skim off foam, add kombu, reduce heat, and simmer, covered, for 1 hour.

2. In a 4-quart saucepan, sauté onions and garlic in oil for 3–4 minutes. Add mushrooms and sauté until mushrooms are cooked.

3. When garbanzos are done, drain, and add to sautéed vegetables. Add 5 cups water, bay leaf, and thyme. Bring to boil, reduce heat, cover, and simmer for 45 minutes to 1 hour.

4. Purée miso in a little cooking liquid. Add miso purée to pot.

5. Add greens and simmer, covered, for 5 minutes. Add lemon juice, to taste.

PER SERVING Calories: 86 | Fat: 2g | Sodium: 111mg | Carbohydrate: 14g | Fiber: 3g | Protein: 4g

Carrot Ginger Soup

Downward gathering energy of carrot root strengthens digestive function. Ginger adds dynamic energy. Variations include adding winter squash, sweet potatoes, beets, or cashews. Adding vegan milk, such as almond or coconut milk, softens the spicy edge of this soup.

INGREDIENTS | SERVES 5

1 cup onion, diced
2 cloves garlic, crushed
1 teaspoon olive oil
4 medium carrots, diced
5 cups spring water
1½ teaspoon sweet white miso
¼ teaspoon ginger juice
¼ cup parsley, chopped

Carrot Onion Butter

Carrot Onion Butter is a kind of sweet vegetable jam used as spread on toast, rice cakes, or muffins. Sauté 5 cups diced carrots and 5 cups diced onion in 2 tablespoons olive oil for 5 minutes. Add water to cover vegetables. Add a pinch sea salt, bring to boil, lower heat, and simmer, covered. After several hours, sweet vegetables will become thick jam.

1. In a soup pot, sauté onion and garlic in olive oil until translucent.

2. Add carrots and water. Bring to boil, reduce heat, and simmer, covered, until carrots are soft, about 20 minutes.

3. Purée miso in a little cooking liquid. Add miso purée to soup.

4. Add ginger juice. Simmer 3 more minutes.

5. Purée soup in a food mill or blender. Garnish with parsley.

PER SERVING Calories: 47 | Fat: 1g | Sodium: 75mg | Carbohydrate: 9g | Fiber: 2g | Protein: 1g

Peas-ful Pea Soup with Squash

Upward rising energy in pea soup supports liver function and holds the promise of spring awakenings. Rutabaga or sweet potatoes can be substituted for squash. Add cooked barley, tempeh, or mushrooms for a heartier soup. Add ginger juice in place of lemon juice for more dynamic energy.

INGREDIENTS | SERVES 5

1 cup split peas, soaked

4 cups spring water

1 stamp-sized piece kombu

½ medium onion, diced

1 clove garlic, crushed

1 teaspoon sesame oil

1 bay leaf

½ teaspoon dried thyme

¾ cup kabocha squash, cubed

¼ cup carrot, diced

¼ cup celery, diced

¼ cup burdock, thinly sliced

Sea salt, to taste

Lemon juice, to taste

¼ cup parsley, chopped

Adjusting Cooking for Warm Weather

Adjust your cooking to create light (yin) meals in warm (yang) weather. To make a dish more yin, use cooking methods that add cooling energy and less flavor, such as blanching, adding less salt, decreasing cooking time, cutting vegetables into smaller pieces, using a light pot, and adding more water.

1. Discard soaking water. Put split peas into large soup pot and add fresh water. Bring to boil and skim off foam. Add kombu. Reduce heat and simmer for 30 minutes, covered.

2. Meanwhile, sauté onion and garlic in oil until translucent.

3. After 30 minutes, add onion, garlic, bay leaf, dried thyme, and remaining vegetables to soup. Bring soup back to boil, reduce flame, and simmer, covered, for 50 minutes.

4. Season with sea salt. Simmer, covered, 5 more minutes.

5. Add lemon juice, to taste. Garnish with parsley.

PER SERVING Calories: 164 | Fat: 1g | Sodium: 39mg | Carbohydrate: 29g | Fiber: 11g | Protein: 10g

CHAPTER 14

"Scentsational" Sauces

Ume Plum Pumpkin Seed Sauce

A delicious sauce can transform the simplest food into a gourmet delight. Serve this sauce over greens or brown rice. Alkalinizing pumpkin seeds (pepitas) are rich in zinc and omega-3 fatty acids, which may promote prostate health. Zinc may also benefit men's bone mineral density.

INGREDIENTS | SERVES 6

1 cup pumpkin seeds, roasted

1 clove garlic

1 teaspoon dried oregano

1 tablespoon olive oil

1 tablespoon brown rice vinegar

1 teaspoon shoyu

1 tablespoon umeboshi paste

1 cup spring water

Combine ingredients and ¾ cup of the water in a blender or suribachi. Purée ingredients, slowly adding more water until desired consistency is reached.

PER SERVING Calories: 222 | Fat: 18g | Sodium: 234mg | Carbohydrate: 5g | Fiber: 2g | Protein: 13g

Guide to Umeboshi Plum

Japanese umeboshi plum is fermented through all four seasons and contains nature's healing essence. Because it is energetically balanced, it is used medicinally to treat both extreme yin and extreme yang disorders. As a condiment, alkalinizing umeboshi plum helps stimulate digestion and appetite. A wonder food, it energizes, revitalizes, and rejuvenates.

Lemon Parsley Sunflower Seed Sauce

This delicious sauce brightens up greens and blanched vegetables. Lemon and parsley nourish liver function to digest fats and oils. Vitamin E and magnesium rich sunflower seeds can support heart and cardiovascular health.

INGREDIENTS | SERVES 6

½ cup sunflower seeds, toasted
¼ cup olive oil
2 cloves garlic
¾ cup spring water
1 tablespoon lemon juice
2 teaspoons tahini
2 teaspoons umeboshi paste
2 cups parsley, loosely packed

1. Process sunflower seeds in a blender and place in a small bowl. Combine oil, garlic, water, lemon juice, tahini, and umeboshi paste in a blender.

2. Chop parsley finely and add to blender and process. Add sunflower seeds and blend until creamy.

PER SERVING Calories: 170 | Fat: 16g | Sodium: 196mg | Carbohydrate: 4g | Fiber: 2g | Protein: 3g

Seeds of Life

Because seeds energetically represent life, all seeds are good for reproductive organs in women. Pumpkin seeds especially are alkaline (high in minerals), which can balance acidic (yin) conditions, such as candida. However, seed butters, like tahini, are concentrated, high in oil, and should be used sparingly.

Basil Pine Nut Pesto

Serve over greens, pasta, or vegetables. Substitute pumpkin seeds, walnuts, or hazelnuts for pine nuts. Cilantro, parsley, or arugula can be used in place of basil. For variation, add sun-dried tomatoes, black olives, capers, lemon rind, coriander, mushrooms, or artichoke for a different flavor.

INGREDIENTS | SERVES 6

¼ cup pine nuts

¼ cup walnuts

2 cloves garlic

1 teaspoon lemon juice

1½ tablespoons sweet white miso

¼ cup extra virgin olive oil

¼ cup spring water

2 teaspoons tahini

2 cups basil leaves, loosely packed

1. Roast pine nuts and walnuts separately in a dry skillet until lightly browned, about 8 minutes each. Grind pine nuts and walnuts in a blender or food processor and pour into a small bowl.

2. Combine garlic, lemon juice, miso, olive oil, water, and tahini in blender and process. Chop basil leaves finely, add to blender, and process. Add nuts and blend until combined. Slowly blend more water or oil into sauce until desired consistency is reached. Store, covered, in the refrigerator for up to 3 days.

PER SERVING Calories: 170 | Fat: 17g | Sodium: 85mg | Carbohydrate: 4g | Fiber: 1g | Protein: 2g

Energy of Freezing

Limit or reduce frozen foods on a macrobiotic diet. Frozen foods are more contracting (yang) than those stored at room temperature or refrigerated. Frozen foods stored for a long time have drying energy, which blocks the liver's upward rising chi. Freezing also breaks cell walls and changes flavor and texture of some foods.

Leek Tahini Ume Gravy

The upward rising spring energy of leeks supports liver function. Beneficial compounds found in leeks play a role in protecting against ovarian, prostate, and colon cancer.

INGREDIENTS | SERVES 6

1 medium leek, thinly sliced

2 teaspoons sesame oil

2¼ cups spring water

½ cup tahini

1 tablespoon umeboshi paste

2 tablespoons kuzu

1. In a skillet, sauté leek in sesame oil until translucent. Add 2 cups water, tahini, and umeboshi paste. Bring to boil, lower heat, and simmer for 2 minutes.

2. Dissolve kuzu in ¼ cup cold water. Add kuzu mixture and stir until thick. Adjust seasonings to taste.

PER SERVING Calories: 25 | Fat: 2g | Sodium: 175mg | Carbohydrate: 5g | Fiber: 0g | Protein: 0g

Role of Gravy

Like a garnish, gravy adds an important element to a dish. Made of vegetables, like shiitakes, leeks, or onions, gravy is more yin compared to protein, such as tempeh, seitan, or fish. Gravy serves to balance these heavy, dense, meaty proteins while adding delicious flavor to a dish.

Shiitake Mushroom Onion Kuzu Gravy

Shiitake mushrooms have been traditionally used by Asian cultures to treat colds and flu. Beneficial compounds in shiitake caps may stimulate the immune system to fight infection and protect against tumors. Serve this meaty flavored gravy over tempeh, greens, grains, beans, or vegan burgers.

INGREDIENTS | **SERVES 6**

6 medium dried shiitake mushrooms, soaked

3¼ cups spring water

½ large onion, cut into half moons

2 teaspoons olive oil

2 tablespoons barley miso

Tamari, to taste

2½ tablespoons kuzu

1 teaspoon brown rice vinegar, optional

1. Remove stems from mushrooms and slice caps. Add mushrooms to 3 cups water in a small saucepan. Bring to boil, cover, and simmer for 20 minutes.

2. In a skillet, sauté onion in oil until translucent. Add onion to mushrooms and broth. Add miso and tamari to taste. Dissolve kuzu in ¼ cup water. Stir in kuzu mixture and simmer for 2 minutes more. Season with brown rice vinegar.

PER SERVING Calories: 40 | Fat: 2g | Sodium: 217mg | Carbohydrate: 9g | Fiber: 1g | Protein: 1g

Energy of Electricity

Electromagnetic fields, such as in electric appliances, have extreme yin energy. Electrons move at high speeds to heat up elements in electric stoves. Refrigeration further exposes foods to electromagnetic grid work. These foods are not as strengthening as those cooked over a steady flame and stored at room temperature.

Leek Almond Kuzu Gravy

Almonds add delicious meaty flavor to this gravy, which is good over grains, greens, vegetables, pasta, or tempeh. A rich source of calcium, vitamin E, magnesium, and phosphorus, almonds can strengthen immunity and prevent diabetes, heart disease, and osteoporosis.

INGREDIENTS | SERVES 6

½ cup almonds

1 medium leek, washed and chopped

2 teaspoons sesame oil

4 tablespoons shoyu, or to taste

2¼ cups spring water

2½ tablespoons kuzu

Nuts and Seeds

The macrobiotic diet includes nuts (1 cup per week: almonds, walnuts, peanuts, pecans, or chestnuts) and seeds (1 cup per week: sesame, pumpkin, or sunflower seeds). Because nuts have more oil than seeds, they need more seasoning to digest them properly. Roasting seeds and nuts balances oil's yin energy so that less salt is required.

1. Roast almonds in 350°F oven for 7–10 minutes until lightly browned and fragrant. Chop almonds into small pieces.

2. In a skillet, sauté leek in oil until translucent and top is bright green. Add shoyu, almonds, and 2 cups water to leek. Dissolve kuzu in ¼ cup water. When water begins to simmer, stir in kuzu mixture. Stir constantly until thickened. Adjust thickness by adding more kuzu mixture or water.

PER SERVING Calories: 98 | Fat: 7g | Sodium: 657mg | Carbohydrate: 9g | Fiber: 2g | Protein: 4g

Caramelized Onion Mustard Gravy

Caramelizing onions slowly brings out their natural deep, rich, sweet flavors. Pungent stone ground mustard adds downward gathering energy, which benefits large intestine function. Serve over grains and greens.

INGREDIENTS | SERVES 6

½ medium onion, sliced into half moons

1 tablespoon sesame oil

3 tablespoons stone ground mustard

1 teaspoon umeboshi vinegar

1 tablespoon brown rice syrup

1 cup water

Tahini, to taste

Shoyu, to taste

1. In a skillet, sauté onion in sesame oil until browned. Add mustard, umeboshi vinegar, brown rice syrup, and water.

2. Bring to boil, lower heat, and simmer for 2 minutes. Add tahini and shoyu, to taste. Add more water if the sauce is too thick.

PER SERVING   Calories: 41 | Fat: 3g | Sodium: 89mg | Carbohydrate: 4g | Fiber: 0g | Protein: 1g

Béchamel Sauce

Béchamel sauce is a dairy-based white sauce used for clam chowder or clam sauce for linguine. For a vegan version, sauté vegetables (carrots, celery, onions) in oil. Add 4 tablespoons whole wheat pastry flour or spelt flour and sauté. Add 1 cup cold water and 1 cup cold vegan milk while whisking. For clam flavor, add oyster mushrooms. Simmer for 20 minutes.

Mock Tomato Sauce

Serve this luscious sauce on pasta, vegetables, beans, or pizza. For variation, use butternut or kabocha squash in place of carrots for a sweeter taste.

INGREDIENTS | SERVES 5

1 teaspoon olive oil
1 medium onion, chopped
1 small beet, chopped
3 medium carrots, chopped
1 clove garlic
1 cup spring water
⅛ teaspoon sea salt
1 small bay leaf
1 tablespoon umeboshi paste
1 teaspoon dried oregano
1 teaspoon dried basil

1. Heat oil in skillet and sauté onion until translucent. Place beet, carrots, garlic, water, salt, and bay leaf in pressure cooker. Bring to pressure, lower heat, and cook for 20 minutes. Remove bay leaf.

2. Place vegetables, cooking water, and remaining ingredients in blender. Purée ingredients, slowly adding water if needed until desired consistency is reached.

PER SERVING Calories: 44 | Fat: 1g | Sodium: 302mg | Carbohydrate: 8g | Fiber: 2g | Protein: 1g

Energy of Reheating

Reheated foods are twice cooked and absorb additional heat. These foods are more yang than those eaten at room temperature. Foods are best eaten at room temperature or just warmed through before eating. To reheat, take out only the amount for one meal, rather than overcooking the whole dish. Add something fresh to balance contracting energy.

Shiitake Beet Daikon Sauce

This delectable sauce adds nutritious flavor to greens, grains, and vegetables. Shiitakes and daikon can help dissolve fats from oily winter cooking. Nutrient compounds in beets may protect against cancer, inflammation, and heart disease.

INGREDIENTS | SERVES 5

1 small daikon, chopped
1 small beet, chopped
Spring water, as needed
1 cup onion, sliced into half moons
1 tablespoon olive oil
1 cup fresh shiitake mushrooms
Shoyu, to taste

1. In a saucepan, add daikon, beet, and water to cover. Bring to a boil, lower heat, and simmer, covered, until vegetables are soft.

2. In a skillet, sauté onion in oil until translucent. Add shiitakes and sauté until cooked through.

3. In a blender, blend beet, daikon, onion, and shiitake, slowly adding cooking water until desired consistency is reached. Season with shoyu, to taste.

PER SERVING Calories: 114 | Fat: 3g | Sodium: 55mg | Carbohydrate: 15g | Fiber: 3g | Protein: 5g

Roasted Squash and Sweet Potato Sauce

Enjoy delectable Roasted Squash and Sweet Potato Sauce as a dip or serve over greens, grains, vegetables, or pasta. Downward settling energy of squash and sweet potato supports the middle organs.

INGREDIENTS | SERVES 4

1 cup butternut squash, roasted

1 cup sweet potato, roasted

2 teaspoons olive oil

½ cup almond butter

2 teaspoons shoyu

2 teaspoons brown rice vinegar

½ teaspoon dried oregano

1 clove garlic, optional

½ cup spring water

Blend all ingredients, slowly adding more water, if needed, to reach desired consistency.

PER SERVING Calories: 303 | Fat: 21g | Sodium: 176mg | Carbohydrate: 27g | Fiber: 3g | Protein: 6gw

Homemade Spreads

Commercial mayonnaise is a high fat condiment prepared with eggs, sugar, and vegetable oils. Instead, use nutritious homemade spreads to moisten bread for sandwiches. To make healthy spreads, thicken sauces, such as Ume Plum Pumpkin Seed Sauce (page 180) and Roasted Squash and Sweet Potato Sauce (page 189), by adding less water.

CHAPTER 15

Dressings and Vinaigrettes

Black Sesame Dressing

Mineral-rich black sesame seeds nourish liver and kidney function, relax the bowels, and support bone health. Serve this dressing over mild greens, like bok choy or cabbage.

INGREDIENTS | SERVES 4

¼ cup black sesame seeds, toasted

2 tablespoons brown rice vinegar

3 tablespoons shoyu

2 cloves garlic, minced

1 teaspoon toasted sesame oil

3 tablespoons lemon juice

3 tablespoons brown rice syrup

Grind sesame seeds in a suribachi bowl or food processor. Add remaining ingredients and blend.

PER SERVING Calories: 131 | Fat: 6g | Sodium: 689mg | Carbohydrate: 16g | Fiber: 1g | Protein: 3g

Black Sesame Seed Tea

Black Sesame Seed Tea is good for hair growth, reproductive organs, constipation, anemia, tinnitus, and floaters in the eye. Grind 1–2 tablespoons unroasted black sesame seeds. Pour 1 cup hot water over seeds and steep for 15 minutes. Strain or drink tea with seeds. Sweeten with barley malt, if desired. Drink 1 cup daily for 1–2 months.

Orange Sesame Dressing

Upward rising energy of citrus juice, like orange, lemon, or lime, balance heavy, oily foods and support liver function. Serve citrusy Orange Sesame Dressing over fish, hijiki sauté, or black japonica or forbidden rice.

INGREDIENTS | SERVES 4

1 tablespoon black or tan sesame seeds, toasted

1 tablespoon lemon juice

1 tablespoon sesame oil

1 tablespoon shoyu

2 tablespoons orange juice

1 clove roasted garlic, optional

Ginger juice to taste, optional

Grind sesame seeds in a suribachi bowl or food processor to make a paste. Add remaining ingredients and grind together.

PER SERVING Calories: 50 | Fat: 5g | Sodium: 226mg | Carbohydrate: 2g | Fiber: 0g | Protein: 1g

The Energy of Oil

Oil is used for hormone production, healthy skin, and lubricating joints. Because oil has rising energy, cook or combine it with salt for balance. Adding oil at the beginning of cooking is more warming and strengthening, and adding it at the end opens the energy up. Raw oil can oxidize when exposed to air, which can cause digestive problems.

Creamy Herb Miso Dressing with Sunflower Seeds

This dressing uses garden-fresh herbs to flavor your favorite salad or greens. Sunflower seeds add health-promoting nutrients, such as cholesterol-lowering vitamin E and anticancer selenium.

INGREDIENTS | SERVES 10

½ cup sunflower seeds

½ cup spring water

¼ cup sweet white miso

¼ cup brown rice vinegar

¼ cup shallots, chopped

1 tablespoon fresh basil, chopped

1 tablespoon fresh tarragon, chopped

1 tablespoon fresh parsley, chopped

1 teaspoon brown rice syrup

1 teaspoon Dijon mustard

In a blender or food processor, mix all ingredients together.

PER SERVING Calories: 60 | Fat: 4g | Sodium: 140mg | Carbohydrate: 5g | Fiber: 1g | Protein: 2g

Red Onion Lemon Dressing

Serve over your favorite greens, pasta salad, grains, or vegetables. This dressing is also good for marinating blanched green beans, beets, cucumbers, or carrots.

INGREDIENTS | SERVES 6

2 tablespoons lemon juice

¼ cup red onion, minced

½ cup olive oil

1 clove garlic, minced

¼ cup fresh mixed herbs, parsley, basil, thyme, or savory, chopped

Pinch salt

In a blender or food processor, mix all ingredients together. If marinating blanched vegetables, allow vegetables to sit at room temperature for 1 hour to allow flavors to combine.

PER SERVING Calories: 167 | Fat: 18g | Sodium: 23mg | Carbohydrate: 2g | Fiber: 0g | Protein: 0g

Boosting Digestion

Ingredients are often included in dressings to aid digestion of oil. Vinegar makes oil more digestible, as well as lemon and salt or shoyu. Eating more pickles or bitter greens also helps people digest oil. Taking ½–1 teaspoon bitter herbs supplement called Swedish Bitters before a meal also helps improve digestion.

Ume Scallion Dressing

Enjoy this delicious dressing over greens, salads, blanched vegetables, or in burritos. Use less oil to create a thick dressing, which can be used as a spread or dip. For variety, chives can be used in place of scallions.

INGREDIENTS | SERVES 6

4 medium scallions, chopped

1 tablespoon umeboshi paste

2 tablespoons brown rice syrup

2 tablespoons apple juice

Shoyu, to taste

½ cup olive oil

In a blender or food processor, mix all ingredients.

PER SERVING Calories: 192 | Fat: 18g | Sodium: 177mg | Carbohydrate: 6g | Fiber: 0g | Protein: 0g

Macrobiotic Oils

Good quality oils (1–4 tablespoons per day, depending on health) support protein digestion, provide energy, and help the body absorb minerals. Use sesame oil and olive oil regularly, about 5–7 times a week. Because other good quality oils, like corn oil, safflower oil, and sunflower oil, are more yin, use them occasionally, about 2–3 times per month.

Walnut Oil Vinaigrette

This salty, nutty vinaigrette is best served on blanched vegetables, such as leeks, asparagus, and artichoke, green beans, or on roasted red or gold beets. You can also season crispy greens, like bok choy, with a splash of this vinaigrette.

INGREDIENTS | SERVES 4

2 tablespoons walnuts, toasted

2 tablespoons walnut oil

2 tablespoons lemon juice

2 tablespoons shoyu

1 clove garlic, minced, optional

1 teaspoon parsley, chopped

Chop walnuts coarsely. Whisk all ingredients together.

PER SERVING Calories: 79 | Fat: 8g | Sodium: 451mg | Carbohydrate: 2g | Fiber: 0g | Protein: 1g

Soaking Nuts

To prepare nuts, soak them 6–8 hours in slightly salted water to dissolve phytic acid, which can block nutrient absorption. Then roast nuts in low heat (150°F) oven to dry them out. Because tropical nuts are more yin than temperate climate nuts, serve Brazil nuts, cashews, pistachios, and macadamia nuts in hot weather.

Raspberry Vinaigrette

Serve this lusciously sweet vinaigrette over bitter greens topped with salty roasted dulse. Or use to garnish poached pears or fruit salad.

INGREDIENTS | SERVES 6

2 tablespoons hazelnuts, toasted
¼ cup puréed fresh raspberries
½ cup brown rice vinegar
3 tablespoons brown rice syrup
1 cup hazelnut oil

Chop hazelnuts coarsely. Whisk all ingredients together.

PER SERVING Calories: 373 | Fat: 37g | Sodium: 9mg | Carbohydrate: 9g | Fiber: 0g | Protein: 0g

Roasted Dulse

Roasted dulse and nori add flavor and crunch to dishes. Dry roast dulse in a skillet over low heat. Stir often to prevent burning until dulse becomes crisp, turning from reddish brown to rust color. Crumple roasted dulse in salads for bacon flavor. Toast sushi nori by passing sheet over low flame until black color turns green.

Basil Lemon Mustard Vinaigrette

Fresh basil brings a sweet Italian flair to any grain, pasta, or bean salad. Other herbs that can be used are parsley, dill, cilantro, and arugula.

INGREDIENTS | SERVES 4

⅓ cup fresh basil, minced

1 tablespoon Dijon mustard

½ cup olive oil

3 tablespoons tahini

2 cloves garlic, minced

2 tablespoons lemon juice

Shoyu, to taste

1. In a blender or food processor, mix all ingredients except shoyu together.

2. Season to taste with shoyu.

PER SERVING Calories: 310 | Fat: 33g | Sodium: 52mg | Carbohydrate: 4g | Fiber: 1g | Protein: 2g

The Basics of Vinaigrette

Vinaigrette contains two main components: oil and vinegar. The ratio of oil to vinegar is 3:1, but this proportion can be adjusted to suit taste. Oils to use include olive, toasted sesame, pumpkin seed, hazelnut, and walnut. Vinegars include brown rice vinegar, sweet brown rice vinegar, balsamic vinegar, and lemon (or citrus) juice. Additional ingredients are mustard, onion, herbs, and garlic.

Hot Vinaigrette for Greens

Colorful blanched vegetables or bitter greens seasoned with hot vinaigrette makes a delicious warming side dish in cold weather. You can also use hot vinaigrette for marinating vegetables or tempeh.

INGREDIENTS | SERVES 6

2 medium scallions, sliced
1 clove garlic, minced
3 tablespoons sesame oil
¼ cup balsamic vinegar
¼ teaspoon shoyu
¼ teaspoon dried tarragon

1. In a skillet, sauté scallions and garlic in oil for 2 minutes. Add balsamic vinegar, shoyu, and tarragon. Mix until blended.

2. Heat over low flame. Serve over cooked bitter greens or blanched vegetables.

PER SERVING Calories: 71 | Fat: 7g | Sodium: 16mg | Carbohydrate: 2g | Fiber: 0g | Protein: 0g

Miso Shallot Vinaigrette

Asian inspired Miso Shallot Vinaigrette is perfect for artichoke or vegetable dip. This dressing can also be used as a dipping sauce for dumplings or spring rolls. Or try it as a tangy spread for sandwiches.

INGREDIENTS | SERVES 12

½ cup sweet white miso
½ cup shallots, thinly sliced
½ teaspoon lemon zest
½ tablespoon brown rice syrup
1 medium lemon, juiced
¼ cup brown rice vinegar
½ teaspoon sesame oil, toasted
1½ cups olive oil
Shoyu, to taste

In a blender, add miso, shallots, lemon zest, brown rice syrup, lemon juice, and brown rice vinegar. Blend until smooth, drizzling in sesame and olive oils slowly. Season with shoyu, to taste.

PER SERVING Calories: 270 | Fat: 28g | Sodium: 222mg | Carbohydrate: 6g | Fiber: 0g | Protein: 1g

CHAPTER 16

Delicious Desserts

Hazelnut Amasake Kanten Parfait with Berry Good Jam

This luscious pudding parfait is refreshing on a hot summer day. For variety, layer crumbled vegan cookies or millet cake between kanten pudding, amasake, and jam. Include additional flavors, such as ginger, grain coffee, fruit, nuts, cinnamon, and vanilla.

INGREDIENTS | SERVES 8

2 large peaches or nectarines, diced

3½ cups apple juice

4 tablespoons agar flakes

4 tablespoons kuzu

6 tablespoons spring water

4 cups hazelnut amasake

1 batch Berry Good Jam (page 228)

Almond Crème Topping (below)

Mint sprigs, for garnish

Lemon zest, for garnish

Almond Crème Topping

Almond crème tastes like delicious marzipan "cream cheese" frosting. Purée 2 cups almond meal, ½ cup brown rice syrup, 1 teaspoon vanilla extract, ¼ teaspoon almond extract, ½ teaspoon sweet white miso, ¾ cup water, and lemon juice, to taste. Use umeboshi paste in place of sweet white miso for sour cream.

1. To make kanten, purée 1 cup peaches or nectarines with ½ cup apple juice in a blender. In a saucepan, add fruit purée, 3 cups apple juice, and agar flakes. Bring to boil, lower heat, and simmer 5 minutes or until agar is dissolved. Mix 1 tablespoon kuzu in 2 tablespoons water. Add kuzu mixture to agar mixture and simmer 2 minutes. Pour into a baking dish and chill in refrigerator 20 to 30 minutes or until kanten is set. Break up kanten into pieces and mix in remaining peaches or nectarines.

2. To make amasake pudding, place amasake in a saucepan. Mix 3 tablespoons kuzu in 4 tablespoons water. Add kuzu mixture to amasake. Stir slowly, bringing to a boil. Simmer 2 minutes until thick. Pour into baking dish. Chill in refrigerator until set.

3. To assemble parfait, spoon ¼ cup amasake pudding on bottom of glass. Spoon ¼ cup kanten on top of amasake pudding. Top with about 2 tablespoons of almond cream and 2 tablespoons berry jam. Repeat layers until all used up. Garnish with a mint leaf and lemon zest.

PER SERVING Calories: 434 | Fat: 16g | Sodium: 49mg | Carbohydrate: 67g | Fiber: 9g | Protein: 9g

Seasonal Fruit Millet Cake

Sweetened cooked millet makes a delicious cake topped with beautiful layers of fresh seasonal fruit. Quinoa, polenta, or couscous cooked in amasake or apple juice can be used in place of millet.

INGREDIENTS | SERVES 8

¾ cup millet

3¾ cups apple juice

½ cup water

⅛ teaspoon salt

2 teaspoons agar flakes

2 cups fresh fruit, diced or thinly sliced

3½ tablespoons kuzu

4 tablespoons cold water

Amasake, to taste

Amasake

Amasake is a sweet drink made from fermented sweet brown rice. To make homemade amasake, add koji (spore) to cooked sweet brown rice cooled to 90–130°F. Mix in koji, cover with cheesecloth, and let sit at this temperature range for 8–12 hours. When mixture tastes sweet, bring to boil, lower heat, and simmer 10–15 minutes.

1. Soak millet overnight in 2¼ cups apple juice. Bring to boil, lower heat, and simmer, covered, for 25 minutes.

2. Pour millet into a 10" tart pan or baking dish, and gently pat millet down with a wet hand to make a crust.

3. To make agar glaze, bring 1½ cups apple juice, water, salt, and agar flakes to boil. Stir to dissolve agar. When agar is dissolved, lower heat, and cook 2 minutes. Add fruit. Mix kuzu in 4 tablespoons cold water. Add kuzu mixture, stirring constantly until mixture becomes clear. Remove from heat and let cool.

4. Pour fruit topping over millet crust. Chill in refrigerator until set. Top with amasake before serving. If using summer melons or berries, pour hot agar glaze or amasake on top of fruit instead of cooking them to preserve freshness.

PER SERVING Calories: 126 | Fat: 1g | Sodium: 43mg | Carbohydrate: 31g | Fiber: 2g | Protein: 2g

Apple and Pear Crisp with Green Tea Syrup

Green tea helps discharge animal food, such as eggs, from the body. Antioxidant-rich green tea also helps reduce cholesterol levels. Steeping green tea in a ceramic pot gives it a softening, relaxing effect, which dissolves hardening effects of animal food.

INGREDIENTS | SERVES 8

2 large pears, sliced
2 large apples, sliced
1 tablespoon lemon juice
1 cup dried cherries, fruit sweetened
⅛ teaspoon sea salt
½ cup water
2 bags green tea
½ cup apple juice
1 teaspoon ground cinnamon
½ cup roasted walnuts, chopped
½ cup roasted pumpkin seeds
½ cup oatmeal or puffed brown rice
1 teaspoon sesame oil
2 tablespoons brown rice syrup

1. Preheat oven to 350°F. Toss pears and apples with lemon juice in a large mixing bowl. Gently mix in cherries and sea salt.

2. Heat ½ cup water to boiling and add tea bags, steeping for 5 minutes. Remove tea bags and stir in apple juice. Add tea to fruit mixture and mix. Transfer to a 9" × 13" baking dish.

3. To make granola topping, combine cinnamon, walnuts, pumpkin seeds, oatmeal, sesame oil, and brown rice syrup. Sprinkle topping over fruit.

4. Bake uncovered for 30 minutes until bubbly and top is beginning to brown. Serve immediately.

PER SERVING Calories: 306 | Fat: 12g | Sodium: 48mg | Carbohydrate: 46g | Fiber: 10g | Protein: 7g

Poached Pears in Apple Cider

Autumn pears are poached in spicy, sweet apple cider broth, which is reduced to make thick syrup.
For variety, add apples and cranberries and purée to make spicy apple or cranberry sauce.

INGREDIENTS | SERVES 6

6 pears
2 quarts apple cider
1 stick cinnamon
1 teaspoon star anise
1 teaspoon cloves
1 tablespoon vanilla extract
2 slices fresh ginger
6 sprigs fresh mint leaves
Orange zest, for garnish

1. Cut pears in half and core. In a saucepan, add pears, cider, cinnamon, star anise, cloves, vanilla, and ginger. Bring to boil, lower heat, and simmer, covered, for 15–20 minutes or until pears are just tender.

2. Remove pears to a plate. Raise heat and bring cider mixture to boil. Cook until mixture is reduced to about 1½ cups of syrup. Strain and pour syrup over pears.

3. Garnish with the mint sprigs and orange zest.

PER SERVING Calories: 262 | Fat: 1g | Sodium: 15mg | Carbohydrate: 65g | Fiber: 6g | Protein: 1g

Sweet Somethings

Refined cane sugar, which lacks minerals, has upward rising energy that is too extreme for regular use. Stevia and agave are concentrated sweeteners that also have extreme yin energy. Healthy alternatives are less refined and more energetically balanced: barley malt syrup, brown rice syrup, amasake, apple juice, and maple syrup.

Aduki Fudge Brownies

Enjoy this healthy alternative to regular fudge brownies without spiking your blood sugar levels.
Chestnuts provide balanced sweetness that is low-fat and high in complex carbohydrates.
For a delicious treat, serve in a parfait topped with raspberry jam and almond crème.

INGREDIENTS | SERVES 12

1 cup cooked aduki beans

¾ cup roasted chestnuts or Chestnut Purée (page 93)

½ cup brown rice syrup

¼ cup raisins

1 tablespoon grain coffee

2 tablespoons almond butter

1 teaspoon vanilla extract

½ cup toasted almonds, chopped

1½ tablespoons agar flakes

¼ cup apple juice

1. Mix beans, chestnuts, rice syrup, and raisins in a large saucepan and cook over low flame for 5 minutes. Put mixture through a food mill or grind in a food processor until creamy.

2. Add grain coffee, almond butter, vanilla extract, and almonds.

3. In a large saucepan, mix agar flakes in apple juice and add aduki mixture. Cook over low flame for 10 minutes, stirring constantly

4. Pour into a cake pan and cool in refrigerator until set. Cut into bite-sized squares.

PER SERVING Calories: 161 | Fat: 5g | Sodium: 14mg | Carbohydrate: 25g | Fiber: 3g | Protein: 4g

Kabocha Squash Pie

This pie is a healthy version of traditional pumpkin pie. For a healing diet, substitute rolled oats or crushed nuts or seeds mixed with brown rice syrup in place of flour crust. Roasted seeds can be used in place of walnuts. If filling is too watery, thicken with kuzu, arrowroot, or agar.

INGREDIENTS | SERVES 8

3 cups kabocha squash

1 cup spring water

Pinch sea salt

½ cup brown rice syrup

1 teaspoon sweet white miso

1 teaspoon vanilla

1 teaspoon cinnamon, optional

½ teaspoon nutmeg, optional

¼ teaspoon ground cloves, optional

1 Vegan Pie Crust (below)

½ cup Candied Walnuts (page 246)

Vegan Pie Crust

Mix 2 cups spelt flour and ¼ teaspoon salt. Add ½ cup safflower oil, mixing well with a fork. Add ¾ cup cold water or apple juice. Shape into a ball. Knead 3 minutes. Refrigerate for 5–10 minutes. Roll out dough and place in pie plate. Shape edges and poke holes in dough. Bake 10 minutes at 350°F.

1. To make pie filling, peel, seed, and chop squash into 1½" cubes. Steam in 1 cup water with salt until squash is soft. Mash and whisk or purée squash and water in food mill.

2. Return squash to pot, add rice syrup, white miso, vanilla, and optional spices. Bring to boil and simmer over low flame for 10 minutes or until mixture becomes very thick.

3. Place filling into pre-baked pie shell. Bake at 350°F about 30 minutes or until crust is golden brown. Let cool before serving. Garnish with Candied Walnuts.

PER SERVING   Calories: 386 | Fat: 19g | Sodium: 103mg | Carbohydrate: 43g | Fiber: 5g | Protein: 6g

Lemon Millet Bars

Sour lemon acts as a tonic to the liver, stimulates bile production, and creates an alkalinizing effect in the body. The upward rising energy of lemons is used to lift people's spirits, calming anxiety and reducing depression.

INGREDIENTS | SERVES 12

¾ cup millet

5 cups apple juice

1 tablespoon brown rice syrup

Juice of 1 lemon

Zest of 1 lemon

Pinch of salt

3 tablespoons agar flakes

3 tablespoons kuzu

½ cup toasted almonds, ground, for garnish

Grated coconut, optional

Mint leaves, for garnish

Agar

Agar (also known as agar-agar) is a clear, odorless, tasteless sea vegetable used to gel kantens and desserts. Rich in calcium, agar helps counterbalance mineral loss from acidic sweeteners. Agar's cooling energy also relieves the heavy feeling after a meal. Because of its mild laxative effect, kanten is recommended for constipation.

1. Soak ¾ cup millet overnight in 2¼ cups apple juice. Bring to boil, lower heat, and simmer, covered, for 25 minutes.

2. Pour millet into a 9" × 9" baking pan and press down until millet covers the bottom of the pan.

3. In another saucepan, mix 2½ cups apple juice and remaining ingredients, except kuzu, ¼ cup apple juice, and garnishes. Bring to a boil, lower heat, and simmer, stirring until agar is dissolved. Dissolve kuzu in ¼ cup apple juice. Add kuzu mixture and simmer for 2 minutes. Pour mixture over millet crust and refrigerate until set, about 2 hours.

4. Slice into squares. Sprinkle ground almonds or grated coconut on top. Serve cold with mint leaves.

PER SERVING Calories: 125 | Fat: 3g | Sodium: 17mg | Carbohydrate: 26g | Fiber: 2g | Protein: 2g

Baked Stuffed Apples

Fillings for autumn baked apples include sweetened pastes (lotus seeds, aduki, sesame seed, chestnut), raisins, rolled oats, sunflower seeds, and walnuts. Flavorings include cinnamon, vanilla, orange zest, or mint leaves. For weakened conditions, steam apples with a pinch of salt without stuffing.

INGREDIENTS | SERVES 2

2 large apples

1 tablespoon pumpkin seeds, roasted

1 tablespoon dried cranberries, fruit sweetened

1 teaspoon sweet white miso

4 tablespoons tahini

Brown rice syrup or barley malt syrup, to taste

¾ cup water or apple juice

2 teaspoons kuzu

1. Preheat oven to 375°F. Slice top part of apples and hollow out the cores without going all the way through the apples. Mix all other ingredients except kuzu and water or apple juice. Fill apples with stuffing. Place tops back on apples.

2. Place apples in a baking pan. Pour ½ cup water or apple juice in bottom of pan. Bake apples, covered, 35–45 minutes until tender.

3. To make glaze, dissolve kuzu in ¼ cup water. Heat while stirring until kuzu becomes translucent.

4. Pour kuzu glaze over apples and serve.

PER SERVING Calories: 340 | Fat: 20g | Sodium: 94mg | Carbohydrate: 43g | Fiber: 8g | Protein: 8g

Sweetened Lotus Seed Paste

Cooked with wakame or kombu, lotus seeds are good for women's reproductive organs. Use sweetened lotus seed paste as filling for desserts. Soak 1 cup lotus seeds in 2 cups water overnight. Remove green sprout inside seeds. Steam lotus seeds for 1 hour until soft. Sweeten with brown rice syrup. Purée.

Faux Chocolate Aduki Cherry Balls

A traditional delicacy, aduki bean paste is used in Asian cuisine to make desserts called "moon cakes," used for mid-autumn festival celebration. Flavorings for aduki paste can include grain coffee, raisins, orange zest, vanilla, cinnamon, coconut, ginger, and nuts.

INGREDIENTS | SERVES 24

1 cup dried cherries, fruit sweetened

Spring water, as needed

Pinch salt

¼ cup raisins, minced

¼ cup brown rice syrup

1 teaspoon almond extract

¼ cup grain coffee powder

Sweetened Aduki Bean Paste (below)

1 cup toasted pecans, chopped

¼ cup coconut, optional

1. In a saucepan, add dried cherries, water to cover cherries, and salt. Bring to boil, lower heat, and simmer until cherries are soft. Drain cherries.

2. In a bowl, mix all ingredients except ¼ cup pecans and coconut. Form into balls and roll in remaining pecans and coconut.

PER SERVING Calories: 117 | Fat: 3g | Sodium: 37mg | Carbohydrate: 19g | Fiber: 4g | Protein: 3g

Sweetened Aduki Bean Paste

Use sweetened pastes (aduki bean, lotus seed, chestnut, sesame seed) to stuff steamed buns or coat rice patties. To make aduki bean paste, pressure cook 1 cup soaked aduki beans with 3 cups water for 40 minutes. Season, to taste, with salt and sweetener (brown rice syrup, maple syrup, raisins, fruit jam). Cook 10 minutes. Purée.

Cherry Lemon Apple Pudding

Refreshingly cool, this pudding is perfect for hot summer days. An antioxidant-rich "super fruit," cherries can ease the pain from arthritis inflammation and gout as well as prevent against heart disease, diabetes, and certain cancers.

INGREDIENTS | SERVES 4

3¼ cups apple juice or amasake

1 cup fresh cherries, pitted and sliced

1 tablespoon brown rice syrup

Juice of 1 lemon

Zest of 1 lemon

Pinch of salt

3 tablespoons kuzu

Mint leaves for garnish

1. In a saucepan, mix 3 cups apple juice or amasake and remaining ingredients, except kuzu and mint. Bring to boil, lower heat, and simmer, covered, 5 minutes.

2. Dissolve kuzu in ¼ cup apple juice or amasake. Add kuzu mixture and simmer 2 minutes. Add more kuzu, dissolved in water, if needed, to make a thicker pudding. Garnish with mint leaves.

PER SERVING Calories: 139 | Fat: 0g | Sodium: 36mg | Carbohydrate: 40g | Fiber: 1g | Protein: 1g

CHAPTER 17

Condiments and Pickles

Gomashio

This condiment (24 to 1 ratio seeds to salt) is the perfect balance of oil and minerals. Sea vegetable flakes may be added to boost nutritional content. Gomashio can also be made with black sesame seeds, which are rich in minerals.

INGREDIENTS | SERVES 16

1 teaspoon sea salt
½ cup tan sesame seeds, rinsed

Guide to Gomashio

Sesame salt (gomashio) is an alkalinizing condiment that aids digestion. It also relieves fatigue, strengthens the nervous system, boosts natural immunity, and increases longevity. Sea salt and sesame seeds are roasted and ground together to create a marriage of yin and yang energies. Store gomashio in a covered jar for two weeks unrefrigerated.

1. Heat skillet over medium heat. Roast salt for 2 minutes.

2. Pour salt into suribachi. Grind salt into powder.

3. Roast sesame seeds until you can break them between the thumb and weakest finger on the weakest hand by rolling.

4. Pour seeds into suribachi. Grind salt and seeds together until they are 80 percent ground.

5. Allow to cool and store in a covered jar.

PER SERVING Calories: 26 | Fat: 2g | Sodium: 146mg | Carbohydrate: 1g | Fiber: 1g | Protein: 1g

Scallion Miso Condiment

This condiment helps the liver discharge fatty deposits, rebalances the entire digestive tract, and relieves respiratory problems, such as asthma and bronchitis. Radish tops, carrot tops, or leeks can be used in place of scallions.

INGREDIENTS | SERVES 6

3 teaspoons barley miso

3 teaspoons water

1 tablespoon sesame oil

2 bunches scallions, sliced

1 teaspoon orange zest, optional

2 teaspoons sesame seeds, toasted

1. Purée miso in water to make a paste.

2. Heat oil in a skillet, and sauté scallions until soft.

3. Add miso purée and toss with scallions. Stir in orange zest.

4. Garnish with sesame seeds. Serve.

PER SERVING Calories: 47 | Fat: 3g | Sodium: 115mg | Carbohydrate: 5g | Fiber: 2g | Protein: 1g

Guide to Miso-Based Condiments

Miso-based condiments contain the energy as well as health benefits of miso. These condiments increase stamina, strengthen metabolism, and improve digestion. Additionally, they enhance beauty, prevent heart problems, and relieve allergies. Miso also removes radioactive elements from the body.

Nori Ginger Condiment

Nori paste draws out soft dairy from the body. Because this condiment is very pungent and salty, only use 1 tablespoon on the plate. Mirin or water may be substituted for apple juice. A dill pickle may be used in place of ginger juice or ginger may be omitted altogether.

INGREDIENTS | SERVES 4

5 to 6 sheets sushi nori, cut into 1" pieces

¼ teaspoon ginger juice

¼ cup apple juice

¼ cup spring water

Shoyu, to taste

½ teaspoon toasted sesame seeds, optional

1. In a small saucepan, bring nori, ginger juice, apple juice, and water to a boil.

2. Lower heat and simmer until nori is a thick paste.

3. Season with shoyu, to taste.

4. Optional: Grind toasted sesame seeds in a suribachi. Mix ground seeds into nori paste.

PER SERVING Calories: 11 | Fat: 0g | Sodium: 8mg | Carbohydrate: 3g | Fiber: 2g | Protein: 2g

Guide to Sea Vegetable Condiments

Nutrition-boosting sea vegetable condiments are a way to increase the healing power of your plate. These condiments are high in calcium, iron, and other minerals. As miracle workers, sea vegetable condiments also strengthen the heart, kidney, and nervous system; revitalize the body; and cleanse the blood.

Purple Cabbage, Cucumber, Celery, and Apple Pressed Salad

Pressed salads support the liver with upward rising energy and are refreshing in warm weather. Any kind of watery, soft vegetable works well for pressed salads. Eat only ½–1 cup at once. Dulse or wakame can be added to boost nutritional content.

INGREDIENTS | SERVES 6

½ cup carrot, grated

½ cup purple cabbage, finely sliced

½ cup sour green apple, finely sliced

½ cup celery, finely sliced

½ cup cucumber, finely sliced

1½ teaspoon sea salt

Lemon juice, to taste

What Is Pressed Salad?

Pressed salad is thinly sliced vegetables lightly pickled with sea salt, shoyu, brown rice vinegar, or umeboshi vinegar. Vegetables are pressed with a pickle press or placed in a crock and pressed with a weighted plate. This method "cooks" vegetables by breaking down fiber, making them more digestible. Because it is lightly cooked, eat pressed salad at the end of your meal.

1. In a large bowl, mix all ingredients except lemon juice. Massage gently by hand.

2. Transfer to a crock and place a plate on top, adding a weight on top of the plate.

3. Let the vegetables sit unrefrigerated for 30–60 minutes or more or until water is expelled from the vegetables.

4. Discard the water and rinse off vegetables under fresh water so that they are not too salty.

5. Squeeze lemon juice over pressed salad and serve.

PER SERVING Calories: 13 | Fat: 0g | Sodium: 209mg | Carbohydrate: 3g | Fiber: 1g | Protein: 0g

Pickled Vegetables and Arame

Black strands of arame add extra dimension to this colorful and dynamic pickle. Make different versions of this recipe using various colorful seasonal vegetables. Arame nourishes digestive function. Purple dulse flakes, which support heart function, can be substituted for arame.

INGREDIENTS | SERVES 4

½ cup celery

½ cup carrot

½ cup red cabbage

¼ cup arame, soaked

1 medium bay leaf

½ teaspoon olive oil

¼ cup brown rice vinegar

¼ teaspoon salt

1. Cut vegetables into thin slices. Place sliced vegetables, arame, and bay leaf in a glass jar.

2. Mix olive oil, brown rice vinegar, and salt together.

3. Pour marinade over vegetables and cover.

4. Refrigerate overnight and serve.

PER SERVING Calories: 34 | Fat: 1g | Sodium: 331mg | Carbohydrate: 6g | Fiber: 2g | Protein: 2g

Process of Pickling

Salt, pressure, and time are three pickling components for pickles and pressed salads. The longer pickles sit unrefrigerated, the saltier and more yang they become. Colder climates require saltier pickles, while hot tropical climates need less salty, but spicier pickles (like kim chee in North and South Korea).

Pressed Mustard Greens

If you like spicy foods, this version of pressed salad adds a kick to a plate of grains and vegetables. It keeps for 1 day, so plan to use it up in one meal. Pungent mustard greens nourish lung and large intestine function.

INGREDIENTS | SERVES 6

1 bunch mustard greens
1½ teaspoons sea salt
Lemon juice, to taste

1. Remove center rib from each mustard green leaf and discard. Slice greens into 1"-wide strips.

2. Massage salt into greens.

3. Transfer to a crock and place a weighted plate on top. Let sit unrefrigerated overnight.

4. Rinse off greens to remove salt.

5. Squeeze lemon juice on top and serve.

PER SERVING Calories: 5 | Fat: 0g | Sodium: 198mg | Carbohydrate: 1g | Fiber: 1g | Protein: 1g

Ume Radish Pickles

These pickles can be made ahead of time and then stored in the refrigerator for 1 week. Because umeboshi vinegar turns vegetables pink, these pickles add a splash of bright pink color to the plate. Other root vegetables, greens, or red cabbage can be used in place of radishes.

INGREDIENTS | SERVES 4

4 small red radishes
¼ cup umeboshi vinegar
¾ cup spring water

Quick Pickles

Pickles that can be made in 1 to 3 days are considered to be quick pickles. They contain more upward, rising energy than longtime pickles and are not as salty. The best time to serve quick pickles is in warmer weather, such as spring and summer.

1. Slice radishes into thin half-moons.

2. Place sliced radishes into a glass jar.

3. Pour umeboshi vinegar and water over radishes.

4. Cover jar with a cheesecloth and store at room temperature for 1 to 3 days.

5. Rinse off the liquid before serving.

PER SERVING Calories: 9 | Fat: 0g | Sodium: 48mg | Carbohydrate: 1g | Fiber: 0g | Protein: 0g

Sweet and Sour Beets

These flavorful pickles can jazz up a plate with bright red color. Sour flavor supports liver energy, while sweet taste nourishes spleen-pancreas function. Serve pickled beets with fresh green salad.

INGREDIENTS | SERVES 4

2 medium beets
Spring water, as needed
½ cup brown rice vinegar
⅛ teaspoon salt
½ cup apple cider
1 medium bay leaf

Herbs and Spices for Pickles

Vegetables may be pickled with various herbs and spices, depending on your preference. Some herb variations include: juniper berries, dill, mint, marjoram, basil, and orange and lemon zest. Some spices to use are: cinnamon sticks, cloves, allspice, pepper, caraway seed, ginger, mustard seed, and nutmeg.

1. Slice beets into ¼" slices.

2. In a small saucepan, cover beets with water. Bring to boil, lower heat, and simmer for 15 minutes. Drain. Place beets in a glass jar.

3. Bring brown rice vinegar, salt, apple cider, and bay leaf to a boil, lower heat, and simmer for 2 minutes.

4. Pour vinegar mixture over beets and cover. Refrigerate overnight.

5. Drain before serving.

PER SERVING Calories: 19 | Fat: 0g | Sodium: 56mg | Carbohydrate: 4g | Fiber: 1g | Protein: 1g

Daikon and Carrot Tamari Pickles

Tamari quick pickles use tamari as the fermenting agent. Shoyu can also be used in place of tamari. Daikon and carrot roots contain downward gathering energy that supports intestinal function. A variety of root vegetables can also be used for pickling.

INGREDIENTS | SERVES 4

½ medium carrot
½ medium daikon
½ cup tamari
1½ cups spring water

Salt Brine Pickles

Salt brine pickles are made with sea salt as the pickling agent. Many different vegetables can be used, such as string beans, cauliflower, or broccoli. Mix 2 cups water with 3 teaspoons sea salt, bring to boil, lower heat, and simmer for 2 minutes. Pour cooled brine over sliced vegetables and store 2 to 3 days unrefrigerated.

1. Slice carrot and daikon into matchsticks.

2. Place carrot and daikon strips into a glass jar.

3. Cover vegetables with tamari and water.

4. Cover jar with a cheesecloth and store unrefrigerated for 1 to 3 days.

5. Rinse off liquid before serving.

PER SERVING Calories: 4 | Fat: 0g | Sodium: 89mg | Carbohydrate: 1g | Fiber: 0g | Protein: 0g

Pickled Mushrooms

These pickles are great to serve with a Mediterranean-themed meal (antipasto). The upward rising energy of mushrooms supports liver energy. A variation is to add green or kalamata olives. This dish will keep refrigerated for up to 2 days.

INGREDIENTS | SERVES 4

1 pound white button mushrooms or other variety

¼ cup olive oil

¼ cup sweet brown rice vinegar

½ teaspoon salt

1 teaspoon fresh dill, minced, or ½ teaspoon dried dill

2 tablespoons parsley, minced

1 clove garlic, minced

Zest of 1 lemon

1. Slice mushrooms thinly. Place in a glass jar.

2. Mix olive oil, sweet brown rice vinegar, salt, dill, parsley, garlic, and lemon zest together.

3. Pour herb mixture over mushrooms and cover.

4. Refrigerate overnight and serve.

PER SERVING Calories: 149 | Fat: 14g | Sodium: 299mg | Carbohydrate: 4g | Fiber: 1g | Protein: 4g

Traveling Foods

Ancient cultures used traditional preservation methods to keep food over long periods for travel or storage. Macrobiotic food that is naturally yang or made more yang can travel over long distances. This includes sea salt and foods that are fermented (aged), pickled, or are naturally dried (grains, beans, and sea vegetables).

CHAPTER 18

A Bevy of Beverages

Grain Coffee

An ideal substitute for coffee, caffeine-free grain coffee is made from roasted grains (barley, rice, or rye), beans (aduki beans or chickpeas), and roots (burdock, chicory, beet, or dandelion root). Bitter grain coffee can help stimulate weakened heart conditions, like irregular heartbeat.

INGREDIENTS | SERVES 1

1 cup spring water
1 teaspoon grain coffee powder
Almond Milk (page 225) or amasake, to taste

In a saucepan, bring 1 cup water to a boil. Add grain coffee powder to cup. Pour water over grain coffee. Stir in Almond Milk or amasake, to taste.

PER SERVING Calories: 11 | Fat: 0g | Sodium: 7mg | Carbohydrate: 2g | Fiber: 1g | Protein: 0g

Roasted Brown Rice Tea

Downward gathering energy of brown rice strengthens intestinal function. Brown rice tea is good for diarrhea, constipation, dysentery, and chronic headaches. It also helps normalize body temperature, particularly in the summer. Add a drop of shoyu in the winter for warming energy.

INGREDIENTS | SERVES 1

¼ cup short grain brown rice
1 cup spring water
Pinch of salt (optional)

1. Roast brown rice in skillet until fragrant.

2. Add water and optional salt. Bring to boil, lower heat, and simmer, covered, for 15 minutes.

3. Strain and drink.

PER SERVING Calories: 0 | Fat: 0g | Sodium: 5mg | Carbohydrate: 0g | Fiber: 0g | Protein: 0g

Almond Milk

Calcium-rich almonds are good for increasing bone density. For a delicious almond milkshake, blend in flavorings like berries, grain coffee, peaches, nuts, coconut, tea, or cinnamon. Optional sweeteners include apples, raisins, maple syrup, or brown rice syrup.

INGREDIENTS | SERVES 3

3 cups spring water

1 cup almonds, soaked

1 teaspoon vanilla

Brown rice syrup or other sweetener, to taste

Nutmeg, to taste

1. Add water and almonds to blender and blend until smooth. Strain mixture through cheesecloth or strainer into a large bowl.

2. Put almond milk back into the blender. Add vanilla and sweetener and blend until smooth. Store milk in refrigerator for 3 days. Shake well and sprinkle a pinch of nutmeg on top before serving.

PER SERVING Calories: 239 | Fat: 21g | Sodium: 11mg | Carbohydrate: 8g | Fiber: 1g | Protein: 8g

Grain Milk

Use grain milk as a soup base or add to desserts. To make grain (oat) milk, simmer 5 cups water with 1 cup whole oats for 1 hour. Strain liquid using cheesecloth, or put grains through a food mill. Sweeten with brown rice syrup. For variety, use ⅓ cup millet, ⅓ cup brown rice, and ⅓ cup whole oats in place of 1 cup grain.

Kukicha Twig Tea

Alkalinizing Kukicha Twig Tea nourishes heart and bladder function. Containing six times more calcium than cow's milk, twig tea helps build bone density. Additional health benefits include burning fat, reducing cholesterol, and lowering high blood pressure.

INGREDIENTS | SERVES 4

1 quart spring water
1 tablespoon kukicha twigs
Lemon juice, to taste, optional

Energy of Roasting

Roasted foods contain warming energy, which activates the body. Dry roasted grains, roots, or teas contains bitter flavor, which stimulates heart fire energy. The process of roasting also adds heat to food, which is beneficial for weakened conditions that need strengthening energy. Roasted grains also absorb more water and become softer when cooked.

1. Add water and twigs to a saucepan. Bring to a boil, lower heat, and simmer, covered, for 10 minutes. Strain.

2. Season with lemon juice, to taste.

PER SERVING Calories: 0 | Fat: 0g | Sodium: 7mg | Carbohydrate: 0g | Fiber: 0g | Protein: 0g

Corn Silk Tea

Corn silk, also known as maize silk, is the yellowish threadlike strands inside corn husks. A soothing diuretic, it helps release minerals to relax a contracted, tight heart (hypertension) from overconsumption of salt or animal food. It can also benefit prostate, urination, and constipation problems.

INGREDIENTS | SERVES 2

2 cups spring water

3 bunches of corn silk

In a saucepan, bring water to boil, add corn silk, lower heat, and simmer 10 minutes. Strain and serve.

PER SERVING Calories:5 | Fat: 0g | Sodium: 10mg | Carbohydrate: 1g | Fiber: 0g | Protein: 0g

Zen Ginger Lime Tea

This soothing tea helps relieve nausea associated with pregnancy or motion sickness. Because ginger promotes sweating, it has a warming effect on the body. Ginger also has anti-inflammatory, antioxidant, and anti-tumor properties on cells.

INGREDIENTS | SERVES 2

2 cups spring water

2 tablespoons ginger, grated or sliced

2 tablespoons lime juice

2 tablespoons brown rice syrup or apple juice, optional

In a saucepan, bring water to boil. Turn off heat. Add ginger, lime juice, and brown rice syrup or apple juice. Steep 10 minutes. Strain.

PER SERVING Calories: 79 | Fat: 0g | Sodium: 20mg | Carbohydrate: 17g | Fiber: 0g | Protein: 1g

Sweet Vegetable Tea

This tea nourishes the middle organs and relaxes tightness from hypoglycemia. Because this tea contains natural sugar from vegetables, it balances blood glucose levels and helps reduce sweet cravings, especially for people with diabetes and candida yeast.

INGREDIENTS | SERVES 4

1 cup carrot, finely minced

1 cup onion, finely minced

1 cup butternut squash, finely minced

1 cup green cabbage, finely minced

4 cups spring water

Add all ingredients to a saucepan. Bring to boil, lower heat, and simmer, covered, for 20 minutes. Strain the liquid and serve.

PER SERVING Calories: 20 | Fat: 0g | Sodium: 34mg | Carbohydrate: 2g | Fiber: 1g | Protein: 1g

Centering Foods

Foods that nourish the middle organs, such as spleen, pancreas, and stomach, contain settling energy that helps center the spirit, mind, body, and emotions. Centering foods include characteristics like round (winter squash, cabbage, onion), mildly sweet (sweet brown rice, millet), and yellow orange color (chickpeas).

Raspberry Lemonade

Water with a few drops of lemon juice provides natural morning energy lift. Luscious raspberries mixed in lemonade add nutrition as well as sweet, tart flavor. Antioxidants found in raspberries protect against cancer and macular degeneration.

INGREDIENTS | SERVES 1

¼ cup fresh raspberry purée

Lemon juice, to taste

1 cup spring water

Apple juice, to taste, optional

In a blender, add all ingredients and mix.

PER SERVING Calories: 61 | Fat: 0g | Sodium: 8mg | Carbohydrate: 15g | Fiber: 1g | Protein: 0g

Berry Good Jam

Berry Good Jam is a delicious dessert topping or spread. To make berry jam, add 1½ cups blueberries or raspberries, 1 teaspoon lemon zest, and 1 cup apple juice in a small saucepan. Bring to boil, lower heat, and simmer, uncovered, until thick, about 30 minutes. Refrigerate to set.

Rejuvenating Fennel Tea

Fennel tea helps promote a healthy appetite and relieve digestive problems. Fennel tea also benefits upper respiratory infections, such as bronchitis, asthma, and whooping cough. To soothe eye inflammation, soak a cloth with fennel tea and place over eyes.

INGREDIENTS | SERVES 1

1 cup spring water
2 teaspoons fennel seeds, crushed

In a saucepan, bring water to boil. Turn off heat. Add fennel seeds and steep for 10 minutes. Strain.

PER SERVING Calories: 5 | Fat: 0g | Sodium: 5mg | Carbohydrate: 1g | Fiber: 0g | Protein: 0g

The Role of Digestive Spices

Spices have long been recognized for their ability to activate "digestive fire." Spices that stimulate digestion include ginger, turmeric, cumin, coriander, fennel, and saffron threads. They can increase production of saliva, gastric juices, and bile secretions. Some can also stimulate activity of pancreatic and intestinal enzymes that aid digestion.

Refreshing Grapefruit Spritzer

This spritzer is a delicious cool drink for hot summer nights. Make with additional flavors, including ginger, apple, lime, lemon, cinnamon, cranberry, pomegranate, and cherry. Rich in antioxidants, grapefruit may help reduce the risk of heart disease and prostate cancer.

INGREDIENTS | SERVES 1

¼ cup fresh grapefruit juice
1 cup ginger ale or sparkling water

Add ingredients into a glass and stir.

PER SERVING Calories: 100 | Fat: 0g | Sodium: 16mg | Carbohydrate: 25g | Fiber: 0g | Protein: 0g

CHAPTER 19

Cooking for Children of All Ages

Noodles with Veggie Kuzu Sauce

Noodles are a relaxing meal for breakfast, lunch, dinner, or as a snack. This luxuriously decadent entrée uses a creamy rich vegetable kuzu sauce. Add sautéed onions and mushrooms for extra flavor.

INGREDIENTS | SERVES 6

2 small leeks, thinly sliced

1 clove garlic, minced, optional

1 tablespoon sesame oil

1 medium carrot, cut into matchsticks

1 stalk celery, sliced thin

½ head cauliflower or broccoli, florets

5 cups spring water

¼ cup tahini

2 tablespoons shoyu

2 tablespoons kuzu

1 teaspoon sweet white miso

4 cups udon noodles, cooked

Parsley, to garnish

Noodles

Three noodle varieties can be prepared seasonally: udon (all year), somen (summer), and soba (all year). While udon and somen are made from wheat, soba can be made solely from warming yang buckwheat flour. Although usually eaten in cool weather, soba can be cooked as cold salad or in cold broth in summer to strengthen the kidney.

1. In a skillet, sauté leeks and garlic in oil until translucent. Add carrot and celery and sauté 5 minutes. Add cauliflower or broccoli and 4½ cups water, bring to boil, lower heat, and simmer until vegetables are just tender.

2. While vegetables are cooking, combine tahini, shoyu, and kuzu with ½ cup water. Add mixture to simmering vegetables and cook 2 minutes, stirring until all is thick and smooth. Taste for seasonings and add sweet white miso if needed.

3. Place noodles in a casserole dish and cover with vegetable sauce.

4. Bake, covered, in 350°F oven for 30–40 minutes until browned and bubbling. Garnish with chopped parsley.

PER SERVING Calories: 376 | Fat: 10g | Sodium: 1434mg | Carbohydrate: 63g | Fiber: 7g | Protein: 14g

Mock Macaroni and "Cheese"

Grated mochi melted into hot butternut squash sauce brings a cheesy consistency to vegan "mac and cheese." A mixture of almond flour, umeboshi paste, and sweet white miso also adds cheese flavor to dishes. Any kind of macaroni or vegetables can be included.

INGREDIENTS | SERVES 5

4 cups spring water

8 ounces quinoa macaroni

Pinch sea salt

1 cup fresh peas, blanched

1 batch Butternut Squash Tahini Sauce (below)

1. Bring 4 cups spring water to boil, add macaroni, and a pinch of sea salt. Cook until done, about 10 minutes, depending on macaroni shape.

2. Add blanched peas. Mix Butternut Squash Tahini sauce with macaroni. Serve.

PER SERVING Calories: 407 | Fat: 9g | Sodium: 14 g | Fiber: 7g | Protein: 11g

Butternut Squash Tahini Sauce

Vegan cheese sauce adds nutritious cheesy flavor to pasta. Cook 1 peeled and chopped medium butternut squash in 2 cups water for 20 minutes. Blend squash and cooking water with ¼ cup tahini, ¼ cup sweet white miso, 1 cup grated mochi, and 2 tablespoons umeboshi vinegar. Slowly add more water if desired.

Brown Rice Crispy Squares

A favorite snack, crispy squares resemble marshmallow treats without the refined sugar. Any puffed grain works, even rice cakes. Toasted rolled oats can also substitute for puffed rice. Add dried fruit and toasted nuts or seeds to create trail mix. Alternate flavorings include almond extract, vanilla, and cinnamon.

INGREDIENTS | SERVES 12

½ cup barley malt syrup

1 cup brown rice syrup

1 tablespoon maple syrup

1 cup dried cranberries, fruit sweetened

1 tablespoon lemon zest

1 teaspoon sweet white miso

¼ cup almond butter

6 ounces brown rice puffs cereal

1. Combine barley malt, brown rice syrup, and maple syrup in a large saucepan. Heat over low flame.

2. Stir in cranberries, lemon zest, miso, and almond butter and simmer for 3–4 minutes.

3. Remove from heat and add brown rice puffs cereal. Stir until puffs are well coated.

4. Press into baking pan and let cool. Cut into bite-sized squares.

PER SERVING Calories: 133 | Fat: 3g | Sodium: 47mg | Carbohydrate: 26g | Fiber: 1g | Protein: 2g

Frozen Krispy Treats

Toasted chopped nuts, seeds, raisins, and brown rice syrup mixed together makes easy praline, nougat, pie crust, or brittle. Add toasted rolled oats or puffed grain and bake for granola. To make brittle, spread nougat on an oiled pan and freeze. For Frozen Krispy Treats, break up brittle and sandwich frozen rice milk dessert between two pieces.

Blanched Sugar Snap Peas

Naturally sweet sugar snap peas make a healthy snack or nutritious ingredient in sautés or blanched salads. Rich in vitamins, they support heart and bone health and prevent the development of cancer. Although they can be eaten raw, cooking makes them sweeter.

INGREDIENTS | SERVES 1

1 cup fresh sugar snap peas
4 cups spring water

1. To prepare sugar snap peas, snap off the bottom and top of the pod. Pull off the thread along the seams.

2. In a saucepan, bring 4 cups spring water to boil. Add sugar snap peas and cook until they turn bright green, about 1 minute. Drain.

PER SERVING Calories: 41 | Fat: 0g | Sodium: 4mg | Carbohydrate: 7g | Fiber: 3g | Protein: 3g

Baked Sweet Potato Sticks

Nutritious Baked Sweet Potato Sticks make a great addition to sautés and stews. Autumn sweet potatoes' orange color comes from beta-carotene, which is an antioxidant and anti-inflammatory nutrient.

INGREDIENTS | SERVES 2

1 large sweet potato
1 tablespoon safflower oil
1 teaspoon mild curry powder, optional
Pinch sea salt

1. Preheat oven to 425°F. Slice sweet potato into sticks ½–¾" × 3" long. In a bowl, add sweet potato sticks, oil, curry, and salt. Toss to coat sweet potato with seasonings.

2. Spread sweet potato sticks onto baking sheet. Bake for 40 minutes, turning every 10 minutes, until they are crispy outside and tender inside.

PER SERVING Calories: 144 | Fat: 7g | Sodium: 102mg | Carbohydrate: 20g | Fiber: 3g | Protein: 2g

Sweet Brown Rice Sushi

This tasty snack is best enjoyed with various ingredients rolled with sweet brown rice inside a nori roll. Ingredients include ground nuts or seeds, sweetened paste (aduki bean or lotus seed), chestnut purée, nut or seed butter, fruit jam, brown rice syrup, and almond cream.

INGREDIENTS | SERVES 6

1 cup sweet brown rice, rinsed

1¾ cups spring water

⅛ teaspoon sea salt

6 sheets nori, toasted

½ cup creamy peanut butter

1 batch Berry Good Jam (page 228)

Sweet Brown Rice

Sweet brown rice is similar in shape to short grain brown rice. An occasional grain, sweet brown rice is higher in fat and gluten than short grain. Because it is richer and sweeter in taste, sweet brown rice is used to make amasake, mochi, or ohagis. The warming nature of sweet brown rice is appropriate for cold weather.

1. In a saucepan, soak rice in water overnight. Add salt. Bring to boil, lower heat, and simmer, covered, 45–50 minutes. Spread rice on sheet pan to cool.

2. Place 1 sheet of nori shiny side down on bamboo mat. Spread a thin layer of rice onto nori, about ¼" thick, leaving ¼" plain nori border around all four edges.

3. Spread a thin layer of peanut butter at the near edge. Spread thin layer of berry jam next to peanut butter.

4. Carefully and firmly roll up mat, dabbing the final edge with a bit of water to help seal. Place seam side down. With a dampened bread knife, slice each roll into 6 segments. Clean off knife with a damp towel between cuts.

PER SERVING   Calories: 290 | Fat: 12g | Sodium: 13mg | Carbohydrate: 42g | Fiber: 5g | Protein: 10g

Pan-Fried Polenta Sticks

A quick snack or lunch with soup, polenta sticks are a great alternative to fries. You can make a dipping sauce with shoyu, water, and ginger. Or serve polenta sticks with Shiitake Mushroom Onion Kuzu Gravy (page 184), Mock Tomato Sauce (page 187), vegetable kuzu sauce, sautéed vegetables, or sauerkraut.

INGREDIENTS | **SERVES 4**

3 cups spring water or broth
1 cup corn grits
Pinch sea salt
1 clove garlic, minced, optional
1 tablespoon safflower oil
Shoyu, to taste

Millet Snack

Millet, couscous, and quinoa are good substitutes for polenta. They make healthy cakes or crusts for pies. For mid-afternoon snack, cook fresh millet with cauliflower or sweet winter squash. Cool. Top with nori condiment. Cut and serve with sauce or gravy. You can even pan fry millet sticks in oil until browned on all sides.

1. Put water, corn grits, sea salt, and garlic in a pot. Bring to boil, lower heat, and simmer, covered, for 20 minutes.

2. Remove from the pot and pour polenta into a glass baking pan. Allow to cool.

3. Cut polenta into ½" sticks.

4. Heat oil in a skillet and pan fry sticks until browned on all sides. Add a drop of shoyu on each stick while frying.

5. Serve with a sauce of your choice.

PER SERVING Calories: 175 | Fat: 4g | Sodium: 28mg | Carbohydrate: 31g | Fiber: 1g | Protein: 3g

Pan-Fried Mochi

This sticky, strengthening snack is made from pounded sweet brown rice and comes in many flavors, from savory to sweet. Pan frying mochi in oil introduces a warming energy into your body during the cold months of winter. If you are anemic, adding oil and shoyu to mochi helps you absorb minerals.

INGREDIENTS | SERVES 6

1 tablespoon sesame oil

6 pieces mochi, 3" long by 2" wide by ½" thick

Shoyu, to taste

2 nori sheets

¼ cup daikon, grated, or chopped scallions to taste

1. Heat oil in a skillet. Reduce flame to low. Fry mochi on each side until browned and puffed.

2. Season mochi with a drop of shoyu or to taste.

3. Cut nori sheets into 4 squares. Wrap mochi in nori squares. Serve with raw grated daikon or chopped scallions to help dissolve oil.

PER SERVING   Calories: 188 | Fat: 4g | Sodium: 2mg | Carbohydrate: 38g | Fiber: 2g | Protein: 3g

Ohagis

Ohagis are glutinous sweet brown rice patties, pounded until grains are half crushed. This is the beginning of mochi. Possible toppings include sweetened aduki bean paste, puréed adukis and raisins, puréed chestnuts, roasted and ground nuts and seeds, chopped tamari seasoned almonds, and brown rice syrup.

Vegetable Pizza

Topped with a delicious sauce and fresh vegetables, this pizza makes a healthy snack or lunch. Colorful vegetables, such as mushrooms, onion, garlic, sun dried tomatoes, corn, spinach, and zucchini are good toppings.

INGREDIENTS | SERVES 1 |

1 medium scallion, sliced

½ cup black olives, sliced

½ cup broccoli, small florets

1 teaspoon olive oil

⅛ batch Butternut Squash Tahini Sauce (page 233), Basil Pine Nut Pesto (page 182), or Mock Tomato Sauce (page 187)

1 slice pita or naan bread

Cooking for Children

Nourish children's upward growth by using less salt. Cook soft, mild-tasting food until children are 2 years old. From 1½ to 3 years old, begin adding salt and texture for chewing. At 2–3 years old, add miso soup with a little seaweed. Cook rice with a little kombu. From 4–5 years old, increase calcium with more seaweed.

1. Preheat oven to 450°F. In a skillet, sauté vegetables in oil for 5 minutes. Spread sauce on pita or naan bread. Top with sautéed vegetables.

2. Bake pizza for 10–15 minutes, depending on thickness of crust.

3. A variation is to add raw vegetables on top of sauce-covered crust and bake 10–15 minutes.

PER SERVING   Calories: 425 | Fat: 16g | Sodium: 1012mg | Carbohydrate: 63g | Fiber: 6g | Protein: 11g

Carrot Salad with Raisins

Autumn carrots are high in beta-carotene, which supports vision health and protects against macular degeneration. Enjoy with optional ingredients such as apple, celery, coconut, cranberries, lemon, parsley, red cabbage, or ginger.

INGREDIENTS | SERVES 1

1 cup carrots, grated
¼ cup raisins
⅛ teaspoon mild curry powder, optional
¼ cup toasted walnuts, chopped
Sweet brown rice vinegar, to taste

In a mixing bowl, toss all ingredients together. Season with sweet brown rice vinegar, to taste. Marinate for 2 hours before serving.

PER SERVING Calories: 360 | Fat: 20g | Sodium: 81mg | Carbohydrate: 47g | Fiber: 7g | Protein: 7g

Grating

Grating is a cutting technique used to break down fiber in vegetables. When pickled with vinegar or salt, grated vegetables become "cooked" by enzymes during fermentation. Grating also activates vegetables, which then carry this stimulating energy into the body to break up congestion. In summer, the energy of raw salad refreshes, cools, and lightens up the body.

CHAPTER 20

Holiday Cooking Celebration

Marinated Tempeh

Protein-rich Marinated Tempeh is a delicious dish for a vegan holiday feast. Or use tempeh in sandwiches, tacos, burritos, sushi, sautés, gravies, and salads. You can even add cooked vegetables and grains for delectable veggie tempeh burgers.

INGREDIENTS | SERVES 2

1 cup apple juice

¼ cup shoyu

1 slice ginger, chopped

2 cloves garlic

1 tablespoon brown rice vinegar

½ teaspoon cumin or ½ teaspoon mild curry

8 ounces tempeh

2 tablespoons sesame oil

1 batch Balsamic Vinegar Reduction (below) or Shiitake Mushroom Onion Kuzu Gravy (page 184)

1. Combine apple juice, shoyu, ginger, garlic, brown rice vinegar, and cumin or curry in a bowl.

2. Cut tempeh into ¼"-thick strips. Soak tempeh overnight in marinade. In a skillet, pan fry tempeh in oil until golden brown on all sides. Add marinade to tempeh and cover skillet. Bring to boil, lower heat, and simmer for 15–20 minutes.

3. Remove tempeh from marinade and serve with Balsamic Vinegar Reduction or Shiitake Mushroom Onion Kuzu Gravy.

PER SERVING   Calories: 511 | Fat: 19g | Sodium: 295mg | Carbohydrate: 56g | Fiber: 0g | Protein: 22g

Balsamic Vinegar Reduction

Balsamic Vinegar Reduction is a gourmet finishing sauce for tempeh or fish. To make the sauce, bring 2 cups of good quality balsamic vinegar to boil. Reduce heat and simmer, uncovered, until sauce is reduced to ⅔ cup. Stir often to prevent sticking to the pan. The vinegar naturally becomes sweeter when reduced.

Roasted Squash Stuffed with Brown Rice Nut Pilaf

Roasted winter squash filled with stuffing or rice pilaf makes a healthy and delicious Thanksgiving dish. As winter months provide less sunlight, acorn squash nourishes the body with many valuable nutrients, such as beta-carotene and vitamin C.

INGREDIENTS | SERVES 3

3 medium acorn or 6 dumpling squash

¼ cup safflower oil

¼ teaspoon sea salt

¼ teaspoon allspice

¼ teaspoon cinnamon

½ cup currants or dried cranberries, optional

1 batch Brown Rice Nut Pilaf (below)

Brown Rice Nut Pilaf

Add this pilaf to roasted squash, dolmas, or cabbage rolls. Sauté ½ cup diced carrots, ½ cup diced celery, and ½ cup diced onion in oil until cooked through. Mix sautéed vegetables and ¼ cup toasted walnuts with 2 cups cooked red japonica and brown rice. Season the pilaf with umeboshi vinegar, toasted sesame oil, tahini or hummus, and nori.

1. Preheat oven to 400°F. Line a sheet pan with parchment paper. Cut squash in half lengthwise and scoop out seeds and pulp. Combine oil, salt, and spices together in a small bowl. Brush squash with spice mixture. Arrange cut-side down on prepared baking sheet. Roast for 45–50 minutes or until tender.

2. Mix currants or dried cranberries into Brown Rice Nut Pilaf. Fill each squash with grains.

PER SERVING   Calories: 564 | Fat: 26g | Sodium: 237mg | Carbohydrate: 82g | Fiber: 11g | Protein: 9g

Wild Mushroom and Chestnut Stuffing

Sweet and savory, this stuffing is a delicious autumn dish on its own or stuffed into baked squash. Stuffing can be prepared a day ahead, covered, and refrigerated. For a delectable treat, form leftover stuffing into balls or patties and bake for 20 minutes.

INGREDIENTS | SERVES 8

1 loaf nine grain bread

1 medium onion, diced

3 cloves garlic, minced

15–20 fresh sage leaves, minced

4 stalks celery, diced

4 tablespoons olive oil

1 pound fresh wild mushrooms, sliced

2¾ cups vegetable broth

Pinch salt

1 teaspoon dried tarragon

1 teaspoon dried oregano

½ cup parsley, chopped

¾ pound fresh chestnuts, chopped

The Basics of Macrobiotic Stuffing

Macrobiotic stuffing contains four basic ingredients: whole grain bread, oil, seasonings, and broth. Dried whole grain bread is the main ingredient; oil infuses flavors of seasonings; seasonings include herbs, garlic, onion, or celery; and broth moistens and flavors the bread. For variety, include additional ingredients, like mushrooms or chestnuts.

1. Preheat oven to 200°F. Cut half of the nine grain bread loaf into ½"–¾" cubes. Place bread cubes in oven for about 15 minutes until just dried out, but not toasted.

2. Preheat oven to 350°F. In a large skillet, sauté onion, garlic, sage, and celery in oil for 2 minutes. Add mushrooms and sauté until mushrooms are cooked through. Add 2¾ cups vegetable broth and a pinch of salt. Add tarragon, oregano, parsley, and chestnuts.

3. Remove the skillet from flame. Add bread cubes and mix. If mixture is too dry, add more broth until just moist but not soggy. Pour mixture into a large casserole dish.

4. Bake, covered, at 350°F for 15 minutes and uncovered for 10 minutes.

PER SERVING Calories: 401 | Fat: 11g | Sodium: 720mg | Carbohydrate: 61g | Fiber: 7g | Protein: 14g

Cauliflower Millet Casserole

This creamy casserole tastes like mashed potatoes and can be served with Shiitake Mushroom Onion Kuzu Gravy (page 184). For a delicious snack, form leftover millet into burgers and pan fry in oil until crispy.

INGREDIENTS | SERVES 6

½ cup yellow onion, diced
1 clove garlic, crushed
1 teaspoon olive oil
1 cup millet, soaked in 3 cups spring water
1½ cups cauliflower, florets
½ cup corn
1 tablespoon tahini
2 teaspoons umeboshi paste
½ cup mochi, grated
1 tablespoon sweet white miso
Shoyu, to taste
½ cup toasted pumpkin seeds, chopped

1. In a skillet, sauté onion and garlic in oil until translucent.

2. In a saucepan, add millet, cauliflower, corn, and millet soaking water. Bring to boil, lower heat, and simmer, covered, for 30 minutes.

3. To hot millet, add sautéed onion and garlic, tahini, umeboshi paste, mochi, and miso. Purée or mash ingredients together. Pour into casserole dish. Bake for 15 minutes, covered, at 350°F.

4. Season with shoyu, to taste. Garnish casserole with toasted pumpkin seeds.

PER SERVING Calories: 309 | Fat: 12g | Sodium: 187mg | Carbohydrate: 41g | Fiber: 5g | Protein: 12g

Parsnip and Sweet Potato Mashers with Candied Walnuts

This delectable recipe makes a great autumn side dish. You can even serve them as a delicious dessert on their own or use them as pie filling.

INGREDIENTS | **SERVES 6**

3 medium sweet potatoes, peeled and cut into chunks

4 medium parsnips, cut into chunks

6 cups spring water

1 teaspoon cumin powder, optional

1 teaspoon ground coriander, optional

1 tablespoon orange zest

¼ cup Candied Walnuts, sliced (below)

1. Cook sweet potatoes and parsnips in water until soft. Drain.

2. Add cumin and coriander. Mash. Mix in orange zest. Garnish with walnuts.

PER SERVING Calories: 117 | Fat: 3g | Sodium: 40mg | Carbohydrate: 21g | Fiber: 4g | Protein: 2g

Candied Walnuts

Candied walnuts are a delicious topping for desserts, sushi, or puréed vegetables. Spread 1 cup walnuts on a baking sheet and toast in a 350°F oven for 5 minutes. Mix 1 tablespoon barley malt syrup with warm walnuts, coating each nut evenly. Spread walnuts over wax paper or parchment paper to cool.

Cranberry Chutney

Cranberry Chutney is very different in taste from traditional sweet cranberry sauce. It can be used as a topping or filling for desserts. Optional ingredients to suit your taste and that of your guests include dried cherries and apricots, raisins, and apples.

INGREDIENTS | SERVES 6

2 cups raw cranberries

2 cups apple or orange juice

1 slice ginger

½ teaspoon ground cloves

½ teaspoon ground cardamom

½ teaspoon cinnamon

1 tablespoon vanilla extract

1 tablespoon orange zest

Combine all ingredients in a saucepan. Cook over low heat for 1 hour.

PER SERVING   Calories: 62 | Fat: 0g | Sodium: 4mg | Carbohydrate: 14g | Fiber: 2g | Protein: 0g

Vegan Eggnog

Eggnog has been served traditionally during Christmas since colonial times. Non-alcoholic Vegan Eggnog is easy to make using macrobiotic ingredients. To make Vegan Eggnog, blend together 1 cup amasake or almond milk, ¼–½ teaspoon allspice, and ¼–½ teaspoon vanilla. Serve cold.

Apple Pear Cranberry Strudel

This recipe makes creative use of phyllo dough in a delicate, luscious dessert. For variety, make an apple tart by layering oiled phyllo sheets in a sunburst pattern, adding apple filling in the center, and folding up edges to cover filling.

INGREDIENTS | SERVES 8

¼ cup maple sugar, optional

1 tablespoon lemon juice

1 tablespoon lemon zest

1 tablespoon apple juice

½ teaspoon ground cardamom, optional

⅛ teaspoon ground nutmeg, optional

¼ teaspoon salt

1½ teaspoons ground cinnamon, optional

2 medium apples

2 medium pears, Bosc or Bartlett

½ cup dried cranberries, fruit sweetened

2 teaspoons arrowroot

10 sheets phyllo dough, thawed overnight in refrigerator

¾ cup safflower oil

Apple Lemon Compote

Cooking fruit, called compote, adds warming energy in cool weather. Add ¼ cup water, 1 chopped apple, lemon juice (to taste), ⅛ teaspoon cinnamon, and a pinch of salt to saucepan. Bring to boil, lower heat, and simmer, covered, until apple is soft. Thicken with 1 teaspoon kuzu dissolved in 2 tablespoons water.

1. Preheat oven to 350°F. Whisk together 1 tablespoon maple sugar, lemon juice, zest, apple juice, cardamom, nutmeg, salt, and ½ teaspoon cinnamon.

2. Peel, core, and cut apples and pears into ½" pieces. Add cranberries, apples, pears, and arrowroot to liquid mixture. Mix to combine.

3. In a separate bowl, mix together remaining 3 tablespoons maple sugar and 1 teaspoon cinnamon.

4. Place a sheet of parchment paper on flat surface. Place 1 layer of phyllo dough on parchment paper. Brush oil on phyllo dough and sprinkle cinnamon sugar mixture over sheet. Lay another sheet of phyllo dough on top of first. Brush with oil, and sprinkle cinnamon sugar mixture over sheet. Repeat with remaining 3 layers of phyllo dough, until all 5 sheets are stacked, one on top of the other. Place a 3"-wide scoop of apple-pear mixture on one end of sheets, 2" from edge and sides. Lift up parchment paper and let phyllo dough roll around filling until dough is rolled into a log. Brush top of strudel with oil and sprinkle cinnamon sugar on top. Using parchment paper, transfer log to baking sheet. Repeat procedure for second strudel.

5. Bake for 35 minutes or until deep golden brown. Cool for 10 minutes. With a serrated knife, cut each strudel into 4 equal portions and serve.

PER SERVING   Calories: 313 | Fat: 22g | Sodium: 188mg | Carbohydrate: 29g | Fiber: 3g | Protein: 2g

No-Bake Pumpkin Pie

This delectable pie contains refreshing kanten as filling for people who are on a healing diet. Serve this scrumptious dessert in place of traditional pumpkin pie or create festive parfait with layers of crunchy seed crust and silky smooth kanten.

INGREDIENTS | SERVES 16
(MAKES 2 PIES)

2 cups toasted sesame seeds

2 cups toasted pumpkin seeds, chopped

1¼ cup brown rice syrup

½ cup olive oil

2¼ cups water

¼ cup apple juice

½ teaspoon sea salt

⅔ bar agar or 2 tablespoons agar flakes

2 tablespoons kuzu

2 teaspoons vanilla

1 tablespoon coriander, optional

1 teaspoon cardamom, optional

1 teaspoon cinnamon, optional

3 cups butternut or kabocha squash, steamed

1. To make 2 crusts, grind 1 cup toasted sesame seeds in a suribachi bowl or grinder. Mix all ground and whole seeds with 1 cup brown rice syrup and olive oil. Spread entire seed mixture evenly to line 2 pie pans.

2. To make filling, heat 2 cups water, apple juice, salt, and ¼ cup brown rice syrup in a saucepan. Add bar of agar and stir until dissolved. Dissolve kuzu in ¼ cup water. Add kuzu mixture, vanilla, spices, and cooked squash. Bring to boil and turn off heat. Pour into 2 crusts. Chill in refrigerator until set.

PER SERVING   Calories: 425 | Fat: 28g | Sodium: 102mg | Carbohydrate: 34g | Fiber: 3g | Protein: 14g

Kanten

Refreshing the body and liver, kanten is a cooling gelled dessert thickened with agar sea vegetable. Kanten can be sweet or savory, depending on ingredients used. Sweet kanten uses apple juice, brown rice syrup, or fruit. Savory kanten (aspic) uses grated corn, grated carrot, and vegetable stock. Serve with Shoyu Lemon Tahini Sauce (page 134).

Millet Cornbread

This cornbread is heart-healthy snack or harvest meal side dish. A variation is to substitute quinoa in place of millet. Eat with brown rice syrup, apple butter, Carrot Onion Butter (page 176), or almond butter.

INGREDIENTS | SERVES 20

2 cups cornmeal

1 cup spelt flour

¼ teaspoon salt

1½ cups cooked millet

½ cup safflower oil

1½ cups apple juice

½ cup Almond Milk (page 225)

1. Preheat oven to 350°F. Mix dry ingredients together. Mix wet ingredients together in a separate bowl. Pour wet ingredients into dry and mix.

2. Pour mixture into 9" × 13" baking pan. Bake for 50 minutes. Slice and serve.

PER SERVING Calories: 180 | Fat: 8g | Sodium: 32mg | Carbohydrate: 24g | Fiber: 2g | Protein: 3g

Mulled Cider

Traditional Mulled Cider is a warm, comforting drink for cool autumn days. Spice combinations include clove-studded orange, cinnamon, allspice, nutmeg, cardamom, ginger, and cranberry juice.

INGREDIENTS | SERVES 8

8 cups apple juice or apple cider

6 whole cloves

3 cinnamon sticks

Lemon juice, to taste

In a saucepan, combine apple juice or cider, cloves, and cinnamon sticks. Bring to boil, lower heat, and simmer, covered, for 20 minutes. Strain. Serve with lemon juice, to taste.

PER SERVING Calories: 114 | Fat: 0g | Sodium: 10mg | Carbohydrate: 28g | Fiber: 0g | Protein: 0g

Mocha Amasake Shake

Flavored amasake makes a gourmet shake that replaces traditional dairy based drinks. To make Mocha Amasake Shake, blend 1 cup amasake with 1 teaspoon grain coffee. Berries can also be used as flavoring. To make a berry shake, blend 1 cup amasake with ¼–½ cup berries.

Weekly Menus for Each Season

The following seasonal weekly menus are guides to help you design and plan meals. Feel free to make substitutions or additions according to season or health condition. Underlined dishes are to be soaked overnight. Use leftover food from dinner for breakfast or lunch the next day (LO = leftover). Condiments and beverages are to be taken at breakfast, lunch, and dinner. Include pickles at lunch and dinner. Dessert for late afternoon snack or after dinner is optional.

Weekday	Breakfast	Lunch	Snack	Dinner
Meal Components	Grain porridge; Vegetables; Condiment; Beverage	**Grain**; **Bean**; Vegetable; Soup; Pickle; Condiment; Beverage		**Grain**; **Bean** or fish; Vegetable; Greens; Sea Vegetable; Pickle; Condiment; Beverage; Dessert (optional)
SUNDAY	Whole Oat Groats; Blanched Collards with Ume Vinegar	Cucumber, Carrot, and Avocado Sushi Rolls; Peas-ful Pea Soup with Squash; Purple Cabbage, Cucumber, Celery, and Apple Pressed Salad	Blanched Sugar Snap Peas	Brown Rice Porrige with Shiitakes and Miso; Savory French Green Lentils; Braised Romaine Lettuce and Fennel; Pickled Mushrooms
MONDAY	LO Brown Rice Porridge with Shiitakes and Miso; Boiled Salad with Carrots, Broccoli, and Cauliflower	Lovely Lentil Soup with Greens; Marinated Tempeh; LO Pickled Mushrooms	Pan-Fried Polenta Sticks	Soft Rice with Barley; Beautiful Black-Eyed Pea Burgers; Sautéed Pea Shoots and Mung Bean Sprouts; Sweet and Sour Beets
TUESDAY	LO Soft Brown Rice with Barley Porridge; LO sautéed Pea Shoots and Mung Bean Sprouts	Udon Noodles; Vegan Clam Soup; LO Beautiful Black-Eyed Pea Burgers; LO Sweet and Sour Beets	Corn on the Cob with Umeboshi Paste	Forbidden Rice with Edamame and Orange Zest; Roasted Wild Mushrooms, Walnut, and Lentil Pâté; Steamed Kale; Ume Radish Pickles

Weekday	Breakfast	Lunch	Snack	Dinner
WEDNESDAY	LO Forbidden Rice Porridge; Dandelion Greens and Onion Sauté	Sourdough Bread; LO Roasted Wild Mushrooms, Walnut, and Lentil Pâté; Basic Miso Soup; LO Ume Radish Pickles	Rice Cakes with Carrot Onion Butter	Brown Rice Burgers; Garlicky Garbanzo Beans; Steamed Baby Bok Choy with Shoyu
THURSDAY	LO Brown Rice Porridge; Purple Cabbage and Collards with Caramelized Onions	LO Brown Rice; Humble Hummus; Basic Miso Soup; Sauerkraut	Pan-Fried Mochi with Nori	Millet Porridge with Vegetables; Luscious Lima Beans and Corn; Sauerkraut
FRIDAY	LO Millet Porridge with Vegetables; Blanched Collards with Ume Vinegar	Udon Noodles; LO Luscious Lima Beans and Corn; Blanched Sugar Snap Peas; Basic Miso Soup	Hazelnut Amasake Kanten Parfait	Mediterranean Brown Rice Salad; Turkish Lentil Soup; Boiled Salad with Carrots, Broccoli, and Cauliflower; Sauerkraut
SATURDAY	Soft Polenta and Peas; Carrot Tops and Scallion Sauté	Pita Sandwiches with Country Tempeh Sausages; LO Turkish Lentil Soup; Purple Cabbage, Cucumber, Celery, and Apple Pressed Salad	Steamed Sourdough Bread; Warm Carrot Juice	Brown Rice Burgers; Aduki Beans, Kombu, and Squash; Bok Choy, Cilantro, and Shiitake Stir Fry

Weekday	Breakfast	Lunch	Snack	Dinner
Meal Components	Grain porridge; Vegetables; Condiment; Beverage	Grain; Bean; Vegetable; Soup; Pickle; Condiment; Beverage		Grain; Bean or fish; Vegetable; Greens; Sea Vegetable; Pickle; Condiment; Beverage; Dessert (optional)
SUNDAY	Amazing Amaranth Porridge with Amasake; Carrot Tops and Scallion Sauté	Brown Rice Burgers; Garbanzo Beans in Mushroom Gravy; Basic Miso Soup; Purple Cabbage, Cucumber, Celery, and Apple Pressed Salad	Pan-Fried Polenta Sticks	Quinoa and Pumpkin Seed Pilaf; Savory French Green Lentils; Kale, Green Beans, and Carrots with Roasted Pumpkin Seeds
MONDAY	Soft Polenta and Peas; Steamed Baby Bok Choy with Shoyu	LO Quinoa and Pumpkin Seed Pilaf; LO Savory French Green Lentils; Mushroom Cabbage Rolls; Basic Miso Soup	Steamed Bread with Carrot Onion Butter	Brown Rice Burgers; Luscious Lima Beans and Corn; Blanched Collards with Ume Vinegar
TUESDAY	Brown Rice Porridge with Shiitakes and Miso; LO Blanched Collards with Ume Vinegar	Mediterranean Brown Rice Salad; LO Luscious Lima Beans and Corn; Basic Miso Soup	Sourdough Bread with Tahini	Mushroom Polenta Burgers; Aduki Beans, Kombu, and Squash; Braised Romaine Lettuce and Fennel

Weekday	Breakfast	Lunch	Snack	Dinner
WEDNESDAY	Quinoa with Corn; Boiled Salad with Carrots, Broccoli, and Cauliflower	LO Mushroom Polenta Burgers; LO Aduki Beans, Kombu, and Squash; Basic Miso Soup; Red Radish with Ume Kuzu Sauce	Rice Cakes with Almond Butter	Brown Rice with Kidney Beans; Beet and Daikon Nishime with Fresh Dill; Dandelion Greens and Onion Sauté
THURSDAY	Whole Oats with Amasake; Kale, Green Beans, and Carrots with Roasted Pumpkin Seeds	LO Brown Rice with Kidney Beans Burrito; Vegan Clam Soup; Bok Choy, Cilantro, and Shiitake Stir Fry	Fresh Berries with a Pinch of Salt	Millet and Quinoa Pilaf with Burdock; Roasted Wild Mushrooms, Walnut, and Lentil Pâté; Sautéed Pea Shoots and Mung Beans
FRIDAY	LO Millet and Quinoa Pilaf with Burdock; Blanched Collards with Ume Vinegar	Udon Noodles in Clear Broth with Sweet White Miso; LO Roasted Wild Mushroom, Walnut, and Lentil Pâté, Sourdough Bread	Pan-Fried Mochi	Soft Rice with Barley; Beautiful Black-Eyed Pea Burgers; Arame with Carrots, Beets, and Onions; Fresh Shiitake, Onion, and Purple Cabbage Sauté
SATURDAY	LO Soft Rice with Barley; Boiled Salad with Carrots, Broccoli, and Cauliflower	Pan-Fried Polenta Sticks; LO Beautiful Black-Eyed Pea Burgers; LO Arame with Carrots, Beets, and Onions; Basic Miso Soup	Corn on the Cob with Umeboshi Paste	Brown Rice with Dried Shiitakes; Black Soybeans, Lotus Root, and Kabocha Squash; Steamed Baby Bok Choy with Shoyu

▼ LATE SUMMER WEEKLY MENU PLAN

Weekday	Breakfast	Lunch	Snack	Dinner
Meal Components	Grain porridge; Vegetables; Condiment; Beverage	<u>Grain</u>; <u>Bean</u>; Vegetable; Soup; Pickle; Condiment; Beverage		<u>Grain</u>; <u>Bean</u> or fish; Vegetable; Greens; Sea Vegetable; Pickle; Condiment; Beverage; Dessert (optional)
SUNDAY	Whole Oat Groats; Blanched Collards with Ume Vinegar	Marinated Tempeh Sandwich; Kabocha Squash and Parsnip Purée; Ume Plum Pumpkin Seed Sauce	Corn on the Cob with Umeboshi Paste; Warm Carrot Juice	Cauliflower Millet Casserole; Garlicky Garbanzo Beans; Arame with Carrots, Beets, and Onions; Pressed Mustard Greens
MONDAY	LO Cauliflower Millet Casserole; Steamed Baby Bok Choy with Shoyu	Mediterranean Brown Rice Salad; Humble Hummus; Carrot, Cabbage, Burdock, and Daikon Nishime	Roasted Nuts; Sweet Vegetable Tea	Vegetable Shepherd's Pie with Millet Crust; Marinated Tempeh; Mustard Greens and Lemon Sauté; Sauerkraut
TUESDAY	Quinoa with Corn; Kale, Green Beans, and Carrots with Roasted Pumpkin Seeds	LO Vegetable Shepherd's Pie with Millet Crust; Marinated Tempeh; Kabocha Squash Parsnip Purée	Rice Cakes with Apple Butter	Soft Rice with Barley; Savory Navy Beans and Wild Mushrooms; Beet and Daikon Nishime with Fresh Dill
WEDNESDAY	LO Soft Rice with Barley; Blanched Collards with Ume Vinegar	Noodles with Veggie Kuzu Sauce; Cauliflower, Portobello Mushroom, and Garbanzo Bean Stew	Walnut and Chestnut Pâté; Pita Bread; Sweet Vegetable Tea	Millet Croquettes; Black Soybeans, Lotus Root, and Kabocha Squash; Veggie Greens Rolls, served with Ume Plum Pumpkin Seed Sauce

Weekday	Breakfast	Lunch	Snack	Dinner
THURSDAY	LO Millet Porridge with Vegetables; Steamed Watercress and Carrots	Cucumber, Carrot, and Avocado Sushi Rolls; Bladderwrack Vegetable Soup	Mushroom Cabbage Rolls; Warm Amasake	Brown Rice Burgers; Garlicky Garbanzo Beans; Red Radish with Ume Kuzu Sauce
FRIDAY	LO Brown Rice Porridge with Shiitakes and Miso; Boiled Salad with Carrots, Broccoli, and Cauliflower	Mock Macaroni and "Cheese"; LO Garlicky Garbanzo Beans; Clear Broth with Sweet White Miso	Sweet Brown Rice Sushi	Millet Porridge with Vegetables; Tempeh with Arame, Shiitake, and Onion Gravy; Purple Cabbage and Collards with Caramelized Onions
SATURDAY	LO Millet Porridge with Vegetables; Dandelion Greens and Onion Sauté	Vegetable Pizza; Carrot Ginger Soup	Baked Sweet Potato Sticks	Fried Rice with Wild Nori; Black Soybeans with Chestnuts; Fresh Shiitake, Onion, and Purple Cabbage Sauté

Weekday	Breakfast	Lunch	Snack	Dinner
Meal Components	Grain porridge; Vegetables; Condiment; Beverage	Grain; Bean; Vegetable; Soup; Pickle; Condiment; Beverage		Grain; Bean or fish; Vegetable; Greens; Sea Vegetable; Pickle; Condiment; Beverage; Dessert (optional)
SUNDAY	Mochi Waffles with Berry Lemon Sauce; Boiled Salad with Carrots, Broccoli, and Cauliflower	Noodles with Veggie Kuzu Sauce; Beautiful Black-Eyed Pea Burgers; Carrot Ginger Soup; Pressed Mustard Greens	Rice Cakes with Apple Butter	Roasted Squash Stuffed with Brown Rice Nut Pilaf; Black Soybeans with Chestnuts; Purple Cabbage and Collards with Caramelized Onions
MONDAY	Whole Oat Groats; Carrot Onion Butter; Steamed Baby Bok Choy with Shoyu	LO Roasted Squash Stuffed with Brown Rice Nut Pilaf; LO Black Soybeans with Chestnuts; Basic Miso Soup; Pressed Salad with Carrot, Radish, and Cucumber	Carrot Salad with Raisins; Steamed Sourdough Bread	Brown Rice Burgers; Savory Navy Beans and Wild Mushrooms; Hijiki, Squash, and Onion Sauté; Blanched Collards with Ume Vinegar
TUESDAY	Millet Porridge with Vegetables; Steamed Watercress and Carrots	LO Brown Rice Burgers; LO Savory Navy Beans; Glazed Baby Carrots; Clear Broth with Sweet White Miso	Vegan Hijiki Caviar; Brown Rice Crackers	Soft Rice with Barley; Baked Kidney Beans with Shiitake, Burdock, and Onion Gravy; Mustard Greens and Lemon Sauté

Weekday	Breakfast	Lunch	Snack	Dinner
WEDNESDAY	LO Soft Rice with Barley; Kale, Green Beans, and Carrots with Roasted Pumpkin Seeds	Cucumber, Carrot, and Avocado Sushi Rolls; LO Baked Kidney Beans with Shiitake, Burdock, and Onion Gravy; Basic Miso Soup	Warm Amasake	Brown Rice with Dried Shiitakes; Black Soybeans, Lotus Root, and Kabocha Squash; Fresh Shiitake, Onion, and Purple Cabbage Sauté
THURSDAY	LO Brown Rice with Dried Shiitakes; Steamed Baby Bok Choy with Shoyu	Udon Noodles in Clear Broth with Sweet White Miso; LO Black Soybeans, Lotus Root, and Kabocha Squash; Boiled Salad with Carrots, Broccoli, and Cauliflower	Roasted Nuts	Brown Rice Burgers; Steamed Watercress and Carrots; Aduki Beans, Kombu, and Squash; Carrot Tops and Scallion Sauté
FRIDAY	Brown Rice Porridge with Shiitakes and Miso; Fresh Shiitake, Onion, and Purple Cabbage Sauté	Mock Macaroni and "Cheese"; Carrot and Burdock Kimpira; Passion Beet Borscht	Pan-Fried Mochi with Nori	Quinoa and Pumpkin Seed Pilaf; Harvest Stew with Irish Moss; Mustard Greens and Lemon Sauté
SATURDAY	LO Quinoa and Pumpkin Seed Pilaf; Steamed Watercress and carrots	Millet Porridge with Vegetables, LO Harvest Stew with Irish Moss	Trail Mix	Brown Rice with Kidney Beans; Nishime with Carrot, Daikon, and Burdock

Weekday	Breakfast	Lunch	Snack	Dinner
Meal Components	Grain porridge; Vegetables; Condiment; Beverage	Grain; Bean; Vegetable; Soup; Pickle; Condiment; Beverage		Grain; Bean or fish; Vegetable; Greens; Sea Vegetable; Pickle; Condiment; Beverage; Dessert (optional)
Sunday	Buckwheat Pancakes; Boiled Salad with Carrots, Broccoli, and Cauliflower	Noodles with Veggie Kuzu Sauce; Vegan Clam Soup	Steamed Sourdough Bread with Carrot Onion Butter	Brown Rice with Kidney Beans; Carrot and Burdock Kimpira; Steamed Baby Bok Choy with Shoyu; Land and Sea Vegetable Salad
Monday	Whole Oat Groats; Mustard Greens and Lemon Sauté	LO Brown Rice with Kidney Beans; LO Carrot and Burdock Kimpira; Basic Miso Soup	Pan-Fried Mochi	Soft Rice with Barley; Savory Navy Beans and Wild Mushrooms; Root Vegetables and Sea Palm; Steamed Baby Bok Choy with Shoyu
Tuesday	LO Soft Rice with Barley; Steamed Watercress and Carrots	Cucumber, Carrot, and Avocado Sushi Rolls; LO Root Vegetables and Sea Palm; Basic Miso Soup	Warm Amasake	Millet and Quinoa Pilaf with Burdock; Black Soybeans, Lotus Root, and Kabocha Squash; Blanched Collards with Ume Vinegar

Weekday	Breakfast	Lunch	Snack	Dinner
Wednesday	LO Millet Porridge with Vegetables; Steamed Baby Bok Choy with Shoyu	Udon Noodles in Clear Broth with Sweet White Miso; LO Black Soybeans, Lotus Root, and Kabocha Squash	Roasted Nuts	Brown Rice with Dried Shiitakes; Savory French Green Lentils; Baked Daikon, Turnip, and Rutabaga with Almond Kuzu Sauce; Purple Cabbage and Collards with Caramelized Onions
Thursday	Brown Rice Porridge with Shiitakes and Miso, Blanched Collards with Ume Vinegar	Millet Croquettes; LO Savory French Green Lentils; Bladderwrack Vegetable Soup	Rice Cakes with Almond Butter	Forbidden Rice with Edamame and Orange Zest; Country Tempeh Sausages; Boiled Salad with Carrots, Broccoli, and Cauliflower
Friday	Whole Oat Groats; Kale, Green Beans, and Carrots with Roasted Pumpkin Seeds	LO Forbidden Rice with Edamame and Orange Zest; LO Country Tempeh Sausages; Basic Miso Soup	Popcorn	Brown Rice Burgers; Garbanzo Beans in Mushroom Gravy; Carrot, Cabbage, Burdock, and Daikon Nishime; Pressed Salad with Cucumber
Saturday	Soft Rice with Barley; Bok Choy, Cilantro, and Shiitake Stir Fry	Fried Rice with Wild Nori; LO Garbanzo Beans in Mushroom Gravy; Red Radish with Ume Kuzu Sauce; Basic Miso Soup	Trail Mix	Cauliflower Millet Casserole; Aduki Beans, Kombu, and Squash; Beet and Daikon Nishime with Fresh Dill

APPENDIX B

Resources

Books

Kushi, Aveline, and Wendy Esko. *The Changing Seasons Macrobiotic Cookbook*. Wayne, NJ: Avery Publishing Group, Inc., 1985.

Kushi, Michio, with Alex Jack. *The Book of Macrobiotics*. Tokyo, Japan: Japan Publications, Inc., 1986.

Kushi, Michio, and Alex Jack. *The Macrobiotic Path to Total Health*. New York, NY: Ballantine Books, 2003.

Porter, Jessica. *The Hip Chick's Guide to Macrobiotics*. Avery, NY: Penguin Group, 2004.

Turner, Kristina. *The Self-Healing Cookbook: Whole Foods to Balance Body, Mind, and Moods*. Grass Valley, CA: Earthtones Press, 2002.

Stores for Macrobiotic Supplies

Kushi Institute Store

This is a good source for all macrobiotic foods, books, and cooking utensils. Look for all-in-one package deals, such as pressure cooker with grains, beans, condiments, and packaged foods.
www.kushiinstitute.org

Kendall Food Company

448 Huntington Road
Worthington, MA 01098
(413) 238-5928
This company offers high-quality mochi, amasake, and natto for bulk mail order.

Rhapsody Natural Foods

This site provides local, organic, unprocessed, healthy, and delicious foods from Vermont. It sells high-quality amasake and tempeh through the web.
www.rhapsodynaturalfoods.org

South River Miso Company

This company specializes in hand-crafted miso and koji made according to Japanese tradition. It carries many varieties of miso, including sweet white, chickpea, barley, brown rice, aduki, and millet.
www.southrivermiso.com

Natural Import Company

This site offers a complete selection of macrobiotic natural foods. Because of its commitment to quality, the company offers foods that are grown, produced, and created by actual families.
www.naturalimport.com

Goldmine Natural Foods Company

This company specializes in organic foods, natural cookware, and home products. It offers top-quality macrobiotic products that support the balance of body, mind, spirit, and life.
www.goldminenaturalfood.com

Whole Foods

This is a natural food store that carries many macrobiotics staples and condiments. It also offers fresh seasonal fish that is closely monitored to meet quality standards.
www.wholefoodsmarket.com

Trader Joe's

This store is located throughout the United States and carries organic produce, canned foods, and dried products under its own brand. It offers many foods at lower prices than other natural food stores.
www.traderjoes.com

Amazon.com

This is an excellent site to buy fresh chestnuts, sea vegetables, dried shiitakes, and many other macrobiotic items in bulk. It offers discount pricing and free shipping with a minimum order.
www.amazon.com

Diamond Organic Produce Distributors

This site specializes in high-quality, farm-fresh organic produce and meals and ships overnight nationwide from Monterey, CA. It offers a dinner club program and organic take-out for healthy home-style convenience.
www.diamondorganics.com

The Fillo Factory

This company specializes in organic natural vegan and vegetarian phyllo dough and phyllo dough products, including whole wheat and spelt phyllo dough. It includes a search tool to locate phyllo dough in your area.
www.fillofactory.com

Eden Foods

Located in Michigan, this is the oldest natural food source in North America and also the largest independent manufacturer of dry organic foods. It offers a wide variety of organic food based on macrobiotic principles.
www.edenfoods.com

Magazine Subscriptions

Macrobiotics Today

The George Ohsawa Macrobiotic Foundation, Inc., is a nonprofit organization that educates the general public about macrobiotics. This organization publishes *Macrobiotics Today* magazine and hosts the French Meadows macrobiotic camp in the Sierra foothills.
www.ohsawamacrobiotics.com

Cause & Effect

P.O. Box 1250
Hinsdale, MA 01235
(413) 623-6645
This magazine contains educational articles and information related to macrobiotics.

Amberwaves and Macrobiotic Path

P.O. Box 487
Becket, MA 01223
(413) 623-0012
Amberwaves is a network of people and communities dedicated to preserving natural and organic grains and other foods from genetic engineering. Their newsletters and publications contain educational articles about genetic engineering, organic food, diet, and health.
www.amberwaves.org

Lilipoh

P.O. Box 628
Phoenixville, PA 19460
info@lilipoh.com
This is a lifestyles magazine for people interested in holistic health, wellness, creativity, spirituality, gardening, education, art, and social health. Articles contain information that brings a new perspective of how spirit shines in life in practical ways.
www.lilipoh.com

Additional Resources

International Macrobiotic Directory

(800) 645-8744
robertcarlmattson@yahoo.com
This directory contains worldwide personal contacts for numerous macrobiotic counselors, educators, and natural foods cooks. It is a good source for locating natural food restaurants that support a macrobiotic diet.

The Macrobiotic Guide

This is an online macrobiotic community and resource for those interested in macrobiotics. It promotes awareness of safe and nutritious food in the United Kingdom as well as internationally.
http://macrobiotics.co.uk

Macrobiotic Lifestyle Adjustments

The macrobiotic way of life promotes a path of healing, beginning from the inside out. It is an opportunity to refresh and rejuvenate yourself and build up your immune system at the same time. Practicing these dietary and lifestyle adjustments starts with intention. Once you set your intention to live in harmony with nature, profound changes will occur. Your dietary and lifestyle adjustments will evolve over time as you move deeper into the process of healing.

Dietary Adjustments

Fresh, seasonal, organic food is alive and full of vital energy. A freshly cooked quality macrobiotic meal eaten daily strengthens and maintains health. Choose from a delicious array of healthy foods and cooking styles to increase benefits of macrobiotic living. Avoid microwaved, processed, and irradiated foods. Include energetically balanced foods, and cook with macrobiotic utensils in a peaceful atmosphere.

Pantry Items

- **Grains:** barley, oats, rye, wheat, quinoa, millet, short-/medium-/long-grain brown rice, sweet brown rice, buckwheat
- **Cracked grains:** bulgur wheat, corn grits, couscous
- **Noodles:** udon, somen, soba, quinoa macaroni
- **Beans:** aduki, black-eyed peas, black soybeans, chickpeas, kidneys, lentils, lima, pinto, navy, split peas
- **Quick vegetables for boiled salad:** carrots, broccoli, cauliflower, etc.
- **Leafy greens:** kale, dandelion, collards, etc.
- **Sea vegetables:** agar, arame, dulse hijiki, kombu, wakame
- **Nuts:** almonds, walnuts, pecans
- **Seeds:** pumpkin, sesame, sunflower
- **Nut and grain milk**
- **Pickles:** dill pickles, sauerkraut
- **Dried foods:** chestnuts, kuzu lotus root, lotus seed, mochi, shiitakes
- **Condiments:** green ao nori flakes, shiso leaf powder, tekka, umeboshi paste, umeboshi plums
- **Hummus dip**
- **Dressings**
- **Oils:** olive, safflower, sesame
- **Seasonings:** brown rice vinegar, miso (sweet white, barley, and brown rice), sea salt, toasted sesame oil, umeboshi vinegar, vegetable stock

Sources of Five Tastes

- **Sour sources:** brown rice vinegar, lemons, limes, pickles, sauerkraut, salad dressing, shiso leaves, umeboshi plum vinegar
- **Bitter sources:** burdock, dandelion greens, gomashio, green ao nori flakes, mustard greens, parsley, tekka, wakame powder
- **Sweet sources:** amasake, apple juice, barley malt syrup, brown rice syrup, mirin, raisins, sweet white miso
- **Pungent sources:** daikon, garlic, ginger, onions, salad dressing, scallions, shallots, watercress
- **Salt sources:** gomashio, miso, salt, shiso leaves, shoyu, tamari, tekka, umeboshi plum, wakame powder

Cooking Utensils

- Baking dish with lid
- Blender
- Cast-iron skillet
- Cheesecloth
- Chopsticks
- Colander
- Cutting board
- Dutch oven
- Flame deflector
- Food mill
- Food processor
- Gas stove
- Glass jars
- Grater (porcelain and stainless steel)
- Knife
- Measuring cups and spoons
- Mesh skimmer
- Mesh strainer
- Metal rack for pressure cooker
- Mixing bowls
- Ohsawa pot
- Oil brush

- Pickle press (or ceramic crock, small plate, and weight)
- Pressure cooker
- Skillet with lid
- Spatula
- Stainless steel pots
- Steamer basket
- Suribachi bowl and surikogi (wooden pestle)
- Sushi mat (bamboo)
- Tea kettle
- Tea strainer (bamboo or stainless steel)
- Wooden spoons
- Zester (microplane)

Bringing peace to your environment can bring you back to center while reducing stress. Prayer before meals is a way of expressing gratitude for the food that was created by the energy of the seasons, earth, sun, wind, rain, and soil. This is an opportune time to show appreciation for the farmers, plants, animals, and chef that contributed their love to your meal. An example of such a prayer can be something like: *I am grateful for this meal, for those with whom I will share it, and for all the sacrifices that went into providing it.*

Enhance your dining experience with aesthetically pleasing accouterments. Use beautiful linens, china, and chopsticks for your meals. Bamboo mats used to cover bowls help keep food fresh. Play peaceful music and remove all distractions, such as television, books, or clutter.

Lifestyle Adjustments

Along with macrobiotic diet, adjustments in ways of living can make a difference in balancing health on all levels. This is *wholistic* living, and goes one step further than holistic medicine, which treats the mind and body through complementary health care.

Wholistic Living

- *Wholistic* living empowers you to assume greater responsibility for your wellness.
- *Wholistic* living awakens and nurtures intuitive and spiritual awareness.
- *Wholistic* living seeks to bring people to wholeness in spirit, mind, body, emotions, and relationships (with people and nature).
- Whereas holistic medicine often borrows techniques from traditional cultures to manage symptoms, *wholistic* living applies the rich philosophical and cultural essences behind these techniques to enhance your life.
- *Wholistic* lifestyle changes can include spiritual practice, exercise, regular schedule, and body scrub.

Spiritual practice

Self-reflection is a way of going within to uncover sacred truths. You can do this through reading spiritual books, developing your intuition, and meditating. Journaling can also help you organize your thoughts and allow you to be open to receiving inspiration. Go on personal retreats to reconnect with nature and yourself.

Exercise

Gentle exercise gets the energy moving in the body, which can help clear up stagnation and build up your strength. Exercises that develop mind-body connection help focus your mind on the body to build core strength and overall stamina. Eastern movement exercises specifically designed to move chi, such as tai chi or yoga, focus on inner as well as outer balance.

Regular Schedule

Living in harmony with the order of nature is the major principle of macrobiotics. A regular set schedule that follows the rising and setting sun adds rhythm to your daily routine. Maintaining regular eating, sleeping, and waking times during the day lessens stress while increasing stamina and productivity.

Body Scrub

A body scrub is a way to connect with your body. Health benefits include improving blood and lymph circulation, removing dead skin, opening pores, and cleansing toxins. It is done in addition to your regular cleansing routine. Begin by filling a sink with hot water. Dip an organic cotton washcloth into the hot water, and wring it out. Starting with your extremities, scrub in a back-and-forth direction toward the heart. Dip the washcloth back in the water. Wring it out and continue to another part of the body. Make sure to do your face, hands, fingers, and feet. For best results, do body scrub twice a day, once in the morning and once in the evening.

Although this book is designed provide an overview of macrobiotics, it is not designed to take the place of a certified macrobiotic counselor and coach. As you integrate the ideas, lifestyles, and recipes presented in this book, you will go to deeper levels of understanding and strengthen your connection with your intuition. However, if you are a beginner, by sharing your process and working with a macrobiotic coach, you can go even deeper in self-reflection than doing it on your own. For the best and most permanent results, I urge you to connect with a macrobiotic coach and take the first steps to your brand new life.

Glossary of Basic Terms

Aduki bean

Also known as azuki or adzuki bean. A small red bean grown in the United States and Japan. Aduki beans are considered to be nourishing for the kidney and reproductive organs.

Agar

Also known as agar-agar. A translucent sea vegetable used to make vegetable aspics and gelatin desserts called kantens. A vegan version of animal gelatin, it comes in the form of flakes, bars, and powder. Use the following conversion: 1 tablespoon animal gelatin = 2 tablespoons agar flakes = 1 teaspoon agar powder = ⅔ agar bar.

Amaranth

A small, round, yellowish grain grown in Central and South America. Because of its creamy consistency, it is often used in desserts or porridges.

Amasake

Also known as amazake. A sweetener or drink made from fermented sweet brown rice.

Arame

A sea vegetable that looks like thin, wiry, brown strands of hair. Along with hijiki, it is used in vegetable side dishes.

Arrowroot

A white starch that is used as a thickener for sauces, gravies, and desserts. It comes from the rhizome roots of a tropical American perennial herb.

Barley malt syrup

A sweetener made from sprouted barley. It is used in desserts, tea, and bean dishes.

Bladderwrack

A brown sea vegetable with a bladder-like pouch that is used in soups and vegetable dishes. It is strengthening for the kidney and urinary bladder, and helps relieve bladder and urinary tract infections.

Brown rice

Unpolished rice with only the indigestible outer husk removed.

Brown rice syrup

A sweetener made from sprouted brown rice. It is used in desserts, tea, and grain porridges.

Brown rice vinegar

A mild vinegar made from fermented brown rice.

Buckwheat

A hexagonal-shaped grain grown in Russia and China. It contains warming energy for cold weather.

Burdock

A black root vegetable that strengthens the large intestine and cleanses the blood. It provides strengthening energy, especially for men. It is used in soups, stews, and vegetable dishes.

Couscous

A small, yellow North African pasta that comes from wheat. It is precooked and then dried.

Daikon

A white root vegetable that dissolves fat and mucous in the body. It comes in fresh or dried form and is used in stews and other vegetable dishes.

Dulse

A reddish purple sea vegetable that is used in soups, salads, and vegetable dishes.

Flame deflector

A perforated metal disk that elevates a pot above the flame to prevent food from burning.

Food mill

A stainless steel utensil with holes designed to mash and purée soups and sauces. An interchangeable bottom allows food to be strained through to remove pulp, seeds, and peels.

Gomashio

A sesame salt condiment that aids in digestion and alkalinizes the blood. It is used on top of brown rice or vegetables.

Grain coffee

A caffeine-free coffee substitute that is made from roasted grains, beans, and roots.

Green nori flakes

Also known as ao nori. A sea vegetable condiment that is used on grains and vegetables and is high in calcium, iron, and vitamin A. It is different from the nori used in sushi rolls.

Hato mugi

Also known as Job's Tears and pearl barley. A wild grass grown in East Asia and Malaysia. It is often mistaken for pearled barley, which is barley that has been polished. It helps dissolve animal fat deposits in the body.

Hijiki

Also known as hiziki. A black, wiry sea vegetable used along with arame in vegetable dishes. It should always be soaked to rehydrate.

Irish moss

A sea vegetable with curly fronds used to thicken stews. It is made of a jelly-like polysaccharide called carrageen, which is used commercially as a thickener in processed food products.

Kabocha Squash

Also known as Hokkaido pumpkin. A sweet, hard winter squash high in beta-carotene, iron, vitamin C, and potassium.

Kanten

A vegan gelatin made from agar.

Kelp

A long, brown sea vegetable that has high amounts of iodine and potash. It is used to flavor broths and vegetable dishes.

Kimpira

Also known as kinpira. A sautéed vegetable dish made with root vegetables, mainly carrots and burdock, cut into matchsticks.

Koji

A fungus called *aspergillus oryzae* that is used to ferment sweet brown rice to make amasake and soybeans to make miso and shoyu.

Kombu

A sea vegetable that comes in thick, wide strips, which is used to flavor beans, grains, soups, and vegetable dishes.

Kukicha tea

Also called bancha twig tea. An alkalinizing Japanese tea made from twigs, leaves, and stems of the *camillea* bush. It is the lowest in caffeine of all the traditional teas.

Kuzu

Also known as kudzu. A starch thickener made from fast-growing kuzu root grown in the southern United States and eastern Asia.

Lemon zest

The outermost rind of the lemon that is grated into desserts and vegetable dishes. It is used as a garnish and to add flavor and visual interest to a dish.

Lotus root

A beige Asian root vegetable that grows sideways in water. It has hollow chambers and helps bind mucous stagnation in the lung and remove it from the body. It is used in vegetable dishes, teas, and poultices.

Millet

An alkalinizing, round, yellow grain grown in China, India, and Africa. It is used for digestive problems and is strengthening for the spleen, pancreas, and stomach.

Mirin

A mild cooking wine made from sweet brown rice.

Miso

An alkalinizing salty, fermented paste made from soybeans, rice, or barley. It is used in soups, beans, and sauces. Miso soup is useful in reducing toxic effects of radiation and excess sugar consumption. Dark miso can be stored unrefrigerated, but white miso must be refrigerated to prevent spoilage.

Mochi

Pounded, cooked sweet brown rice made into cakes. It can be used in desserts, bean and vegetable dishes, soups, and sauces. It is also good on its own pan fried, baked, or made into waffles. Contracting, pounding energy in mochi strengthens the downward energy of the intestines.

Natto:

Traditional Japanese fermented soybean staple, often eaten at breakfast. It has a stringy consistency, along with strong smell and taste. Rich in vitamin K2, natto has many health benefits, including preventing osteo-porosis in postmenopausal women and reducing blood clots and heart attacks.

Nishime

Also know as waterless cooking. A vegeta-ble stew made in a heavy pot with very little water to retain vitamins and flavors.

Nori

A sea vegetable pressed into sheets used in making sushi. Untoasted nori is black in color, which changes to green when it is toasted.

Ohagi

Glutinous, pounded sweet brown rice patties, which are the beginning of making mochi. Ohagis can be rolled in various toppings, like nuts, aduki bean paste, or nori.

Ohsawa pot

A ceramic or glass pot with a lid that is used inside a pressure cooker to cook grains and beans. The Ohsawa pot is placed in water inside the pressure cooker, which is then covered and brought to pressure. Because the Ohsawa pot is placed in water and away from the heat source, the food is steamed and becomes richer and creamier than with normal pressure cooking.

Quinoa

A small, round yellowish grain grown in the Andes. It is high in protein and must be rinsed thoroughly to remove the bitter tannin coating.

Sea palm

A brown sea vegetable having a shape similar to a palm tree. The ridged blades are used in salads and vegetable dishes.

Seitan

Wheat gluten that is used as a protein substi-tute for meat.

Shiitake

A kind of mushroom that comes fresh or dried. It is used to flavor soups, gravies, and vegetable dishes. It can be made into tea to dissolve excess animal fat deposits in the body.

Shiso

Red beefsteak leaves that are used to pickle umeboshi plums.

Shoyu

A Japanese soy sauce that is used to season vegetable and bean dishes.

Soba

Thin noodles made from buckwheat flour or a mixture of buckwheat and whole wheat flour. Usually used in soups and vegetable dishes, soba is warming in the winter.

Spelt:

An ancient variety of wheat. Spelt has higher protein content than wheat and is more easily digestible. Used as a wheat substitution, spelt can be tolerated by those with wheat allergies.

Suribachi:

A serrated ceramic mortar used with a surikogi to grind spices, seeds, and other ingredients into powder to make sauces and condiments. It is used for making gomashio condiment. Unlike a high-speed modern electric blender or food processor, a suribachi and surikogi, like a traditional mortar and pestle, adds a calming, rustic quality to the energy of the food.

Surikogi

A wooden pestle used with a suribachi bowl.

Sweet brown rice vinegar

A sweet vinegar made from sweet brown rice that can be used in place of balsamic vinegar or a mixture of sweetener (mirin, apple juice, or brown rice syrup) and brown rice vinegar.

Tamari

Soy sauce made without wheat. It is the by-product of miso making and is more yang than shoyu.

Tahini

A seed butter made from ground sesame seeds. It is used to make sauces, gravies, vegetable dishes, and desserts.

Tekka

A dark, salty condiment made from roasted root vegetables (burdock, lotus root, carrot, and ginger) cooked with miso. It is strengthening and alkalinizing.

Tempeh

A fermented Indonesian protein substitute made with soybeans and a fungus starter called *rhizopus oligosporus*. If homemade, it can be a source of vitamin B12.

Udon

Japanese noodles made from whole wheat flour or a mixture of whole wheat flour and white flour. These noodles are used to make soups, salads, and vegetable dishes.

Umeboshi plum

A red, pickled Japanese plum that is used in cooking to season grains, beans, sauces, and vegetable dishes or on its own as a pickle. Umeboshi paste is made from umeboshi plums and is more concentrated (salty), and not as medicinal.

Umeboshi vinegar

Vinegar that is the byproduct of pickling umeboshi plums. Its salty and sour taste flavors grains, sauces, dressings, and vegetable dishes.

Wakame

A long, thin sea vegetable that is used to flavor the daily miso soup, other soups, and beans.

Yang

One of two fundamental life force energies. In relation to something else, yang has the tendency of contraction, density, heat, and other qualities. Yang energy has a tendency to condense and go inward as in compact grains (brown rice, buckwheat, and millet), roots, and salt. Its complementary opposite energy is yin.

Yin

Refers to one of two fundamental life force energies. Relative to something else, yin has the tendency of expansion, lightness, cold, and other qualities. Yin energy has a tendency to expand upward and outward as in large grains (corn, oats, and wheat), fruits, and leafy greens. Its complementary antagonistic energy is yang.

Index

We Have EVERYTHING® on Anything!

With more than 19 million copies sold, the Everything® series has become one of America's favorite resources for solving problems, learning new skills, and organizing lives. Our brand is not only recognizable—it's also welcomed.

The series is a hand-in-hand partner for people who are ready to tackle new subjects—like you!

For more information on the Everything® series, please visit *www.adamsmedia.com*

The Everything® list spans a wide range of subjects, with more than 500 titles covering 25 different categories:

Business	History	Reference
Careers	Home Improvement	Religion
Children's Storybooks	Everything Kids	Self-Help
Computers	Languages	Sports & Fitness
Cooking	Music	Travel
Crafts and Hobbies	New Age	Wedding
Education/Schools	Parenting	Writing
Games and Puzzles	Personal Finance	
Health	Pets	